D1766571

Maxillofacial Care

Maxillofacial Care

Edited by

Michael Perry FRCS, FDS, BSc

Senior Registrar in Oral and Maxillofacial Surgery,
The Queen Victoria Hospital NHS Trust, East Grinstead, West Sussex, UK

Caroline Evans RGN

Clinical Support Nurse, Plastic Surgery, Canadian Wing,
The Queen Victoria Hospital NHS Trust, East Grinstead, West Sussex, UK

Krys Peel RGN

Staff Nurse, Plastic Surgery, Burns and Maxillofacial Dressing Clinic,
The Queen Victoria Hospital NHS Trust, East Grinstead, West Sussex, UK

A member of the Hodder Headline Group
LONDON • SYDNEY • AUCKLAND

First published in Great Britain in 1999 by
Arnold, a member of the Hodder Headline Group,
338 Euston Road, London NW1 3BH

http://www.arnoldpublishers.com

British Library Cataloguing in Publication Data
A catalogue record for this book is available from the British Library

ISBN 0 340 71893 5

1 2 3 4 5 6 7 8 9 10

Commissioning Editor: Cathy Peck
Production Editor: Rada Radojicic
Production Controller: Priya Gohil
Cover Design: Richard Kwan

Typeset in 10/12 pt Palatino by
Phoenix Photosetting, Chatham, Kent
Printed in Great Britain by St Edmundsbury Press, Suffolk
Bound in Great Britain by J. W. Arrowsmith Ltd, Bristol

What do you think about this book? Or any other Arnold title?
Please send your comments to feedback.arnold@hodder.co.uk

Contents

List of contributors

Lesley Boys RGN
Senior Clinical Nurse Specialist, Pain Relief Unit, Kings College Hospital, London

Jo Kerr RGN, SEN, ENB 997/8
Clinical Support Nurse, Head and Neck Team, Maxillofacial Unit, The Queen Victoria Hospital NHS Trust, East Grinstead, West Sussex

Sharon Maddix ABDSA, FETC
Senior DSA, Maxillofacial Unit, Kings College Hospital, London

Janet Powell RGN
Manager-Practitioner, Day-Surgery Unit, Bexhill Hospital, Bexhill-on-Sea, East Sussex

Brooke M. Quinteros DipCSLT RegMRCSLT
Speech and Language Therapy Unit, The Queen Victoria Hospital NHS Trust, East Grinstead, West Sussex

Christine van der Valk SRN ENB 998 NVQ Assessor
Staff Nurse, Russell Davies Unit, The Queen Victoria Hospital NHS Trust, East Grinstead, West Sussex

Sally Wharnsby RGN RSCN ENB 264 Dip Prof Studies Child Protection
Sister, Paediatric Unit, The Queen Victoria Hospital NHS Trust, East Grinstead, West Sussex

Preface

Arguably the head and neck represents one of the most complex regions in the body, not only anatomically, but also in the diversity of highly specialized functions that it carries out. The diagnosis and treatment of diseases involving the head and neck can therefore be stimulating, challenging and sometimes frustrating!

Over the years head and neck surgery has evolved to such an extent that it is now becoming recognized as a specialty in its own right. As such, a variety of disciplines have come to lay claim on this anatomical region, including otorhinolaryngology (ENT), plastic surgery and, of course, oral and maxillofacial surgery (OMFS). Each has developed with its own strengths and weaknesses, and all have contributed to the development of the specialty as a whole. However, a fully comprehensive head and neck service requires expertise not only from each of these disciplines, but also from allied specialties such as speech and language therapy, restorative and prosthodontic dentistry and maxillofacial technicians, to name just a few.

During the two World Wars large numbers of casualties with extensive facial injuries required urgent initial treatment and later secondary reconstruction. Varaztad Kazanjian and Harold Gilles are often cited for their innovative work in this field, and are credited with laying the foundations for maxillofacial surgery. In the UK, maxillofacial surgery (also known as oral and maxillofacial surgery, oral surgery, and oral and facial surgery) progressed with the foundation of the 'Oral Surgery Club' by Rupert Sutton Taylor in the 1930s. At that time it was essentially a subspecialty of dentistry. However, with rapid expansion of the specialty, coupled with major advances in knowledge, technology and surgical techniques, the specialty has since undergone radical change. The scope of maxillofacial surgery has expanded accordingly, as this book will hopefully illustrate. Too many colleagues, departments and administrators are still woefully unaware of the breadth and depth of work currently undertaken and all that can be offered to medical and surgical colleagues. Although 'dental' problems still form a significant part of the workload and therefore require dental-based specialist knowledge, facial trauma, head and neck cancer, diseases of the salivary glands, cranial base surgery and cleft lip and palate are now frequently managed in most maxillofacial units. Expertise in the management of pain and anxiety and safe delivery of out-patient sedation is also essential.

Today's maxillofacial trainee must be medically and dentally qualified and undergo structured higher training in both surgery (FRCS/AFRCS/MRCS) and dentistry (FDS/MFDS). This background provides a sound foundation in the understanding of surgical diseases of the mouth, neck, face and jaws, and a unique ability to address both hard and soft tissue deformities.

Surgical and non-surgical diseases of the head and neck and their management are often poorly taught and are generally 'picked up' by undergraduates and junior staff. Only those who are fortunate enough to be attached to a dynamic head and neck unit have an opportunity to appreciate the range and complexity of surgical care that is available. The aim of this book is therefore to give a broad overview of many of the conditions that are commonly seen in maxillofacial practice, and the management of those conditions. This book is not designed to be prescriptive or dogmatic, but rather we have tried to outline general principles of diagnosis and management. It is acknowledged that some aspects of practice do vary from unit to unit (e.g. drug protocols and fracture management). In addition, many diagnostic and treatment approaches will change as advances in techniques and research create new opportunities.

We hope that all those involved in the care of patients with diseases of the mouth, neck, face and jaws, whether they be nurses, doctors, dentists or speech and language therapists, will find this book of value and help to remove much of the mystique that has surrounded this fascinating speciality. Much of its content will also be invaluable to dental and medical students preparing for undergraduate final examinations.

Michael Perry
Caroline Evans
Krys Peel

Acknowledgements

I would like to express my sincere appreciation to my trainers and colleagues who have inspired me and from whom I have learned so much. To date my training has involved attachments in East Grinstead, Kings College Hospital London, Leeds, Sunderland and York, and I am grateful to my consultant and senior colleagues, all of whom have contributed to my understanding and experience and have maintained my enthusiasm. Without their support and teaching this book would not have been possible.

I would also like to thank Mr Peter Ayliffe, currently a senior registrar in maxillofacial surgery, for providing me with many of the photographs used throughout the text.

Finally I would like to thank Mrs Barbara Bradford, who has taken on the unenviable task of preparing the text.

Michael Perry

Assessment, admission and discharge of patients undergoing head and neck surgery

Michael Perry and Caroline Evans

Emergency surgery
Medical assessment
Nutritional assessment
Deep vein thrombosis (DVT)
Steroids in surgery
Stress ulceration
Surgery in the elderly
Facial disfigurement
Admission
Discharge home

A significant number of patients undergoing head and neck surgery are middle-aged or elderly, and may have coexisting medical problems, social problems or other complicating factors. This chapter outlines some of the more common problems encountered and how these should be assessed and dealt with pre-operatively.

Complicating factors are most commonly seen in patients undergoing surgery for cancer, many of whom have a history of smoking and/or alcohol abuse. Younger patients may also have coexisting medical problems that complicate treatment (e.g. diabetes, asthma, haemophilia). Trauma patients require thorough assessment to exclude other injuries which may preclude urgent surgery (e.g. head injury, cervical spine injury) (Box 1.1).

BOX 1.1 Common problems in maxillofacial patients

- Elderly
- Smoking
- Alcohol abuse
- Ischaemic heart disease
- Respiratory disease (e.g. chronic obstructive airway disease)
- Diabetes
- Malnutrition
- Blood disorders (e.g. haemophilia, sickle cell anaemia)
- Head/facial injury
- Cervical spine/multiple injuries
- Social deprivation

In addition, for many patients, admission to hospital for surgery, whether it is planned or an emergency, will be a traumatic event in their life, even if the surgery is considered to be relatively minor. Many patients have preconceived ideas about what the experience will be like, often based on media stories or descriptions by friends or relatives who have been in hospital. These expectations are often inaccurate, and consequently some patients have unnecessary fears. In addition, fear of the unknown is also a source of much anxiety. It is now widely accepted that good-quality information given to patients pre-operatively aids their recovery post-operatively. Providing such information can alleviate anxiety and thus reduce post-operative pain.

All patients therefore need a thorough medical and social evaluation either on admission, if their condition is acute, or on an out-patient basis. In this way those factors which may have an effect on treatment may be identified early and the patient's condition improved before surgery.

Many routine admissions are fit and well, requiring only minimal 'work-up', usually on the day of admission. However, in those patients for whom recovery and rehabilitation are likely to be prolonged (e.g. cases of debilitating disease, self-neglect, or following major surgery), early referral to allied specialists *prior* to surgery is essential. This should not only be medical, but should also involve where necessary the early participation of physiotherapists, dietitians, speech therapists and social services. Staff must also anticipate the need for any precautionary measures in the peri-operative and post-operative period (Box 1.2).

BOX 1.2 Assessment considerations

- Medical
- Nutritional support

- Deep vein thrombosis (DVT) prophylaxis
- Steroid cover
- Antibiotic cover (ABC)
- Stress ulcer prophylaxis
- Effective pain relief
- Social circumstances
- *Pre-operative* assessment by physiotherapists, dietitians, speech therapists and social services

Emergency surgery

Whereas patients who are undergoing elective surgery can be pre-assessed in good time, those requiring emergency surgery do not have this luxury, and can only be rendered as fit as possible within the time allowed, depending on the degree of urgency. Relatively few maxillofacial emergencies need *immediate* intervention (see Chapter 10 on maxillofacial emergencies), and most can be delayed for at least a few hours so that medical treatment is possible. In selected cases some patients may benefit from a brief period of intensive management on a high-dependency unit (HDU) or intensive-care unit (ICU). In all cases early anaesthetist input is essential, particularly for those patients with potential airway hazards.

Medical assessment

This includes:

- history;
- examination;
- special investigations.

BOX 1.3   Clinical history

- Presenting complaint
- History of presenting complaint
- Past medical/surgical history
- Drug history
- Allergies
- Systems enquiry
- Social/family history
- Pregnancy?

The purpose of history-taking is to establish the diagnosis, to determine the need for treatment and to assess the patient's general health in relation to 'fitness for surgery'. Coexisting medical problems not necessarily complicating anaesthesia also need to be identified (e.g. glaucoma, arthritis), especially where in-patient stay is expected to be prolonged. The past medical history must include any history of myocardial infarction, high blood pressure, rheumatic fever, diabetes, epilepsy, tuberculosis, jaundice, hepatitis, other infectious diseases, 'bleeding' problems and asthma. All patients need to be asked about allergies to medications, and in female patients of childbearing age pregnancy must always be considered.

The family history may sometimes indicate potential risks from anaesthesia, and patients should be asked about a history of malignant hyperpyrexia, porphyria and, if of non-European decent, sickle cell disease. People in certain occupations may be exposed to hazards which can produce respiratory disease. These include cancers (e.g. asbestos workers), infections (e.g. bird breeders), asthma (e.g. painters), pneumoconiosis (e.g. coal miners) and allergic alveolitis (e.g. farmers). Home circumstances may provide an indication of what support services will be required following discharge.

Routine investigations

All patients must have their temperature, pulse and blood pressure measured on admission. Urine analysis should be carried out, assessing for glucose or ketones (diabetes), protein (renal disease, especially infection), blood (infection or tumour), bilirubin (liver disorders) and urobilinogen (jaundice). Not all patients require blood analysis; this depends on the patient's clinical condition and the operation proposed.

Cardiorespiratory assessment

BOX 1.4 Symptoms and risk factors

Symptoms of cardiorespiratory disease

- Chest pain
- Angina
- Shortness of breath associated with exercise, cold or after eating
- Orthopnoea
- Paroxysmal nocturnal dyspnoea (sudden shortness of breath at night-time)
- Nocturnal cough
- Ankle swelling
- Claudication (calf pain on walking, relieved by rest)
- Sputum production
- Wheeze

Risk factors for cardiac disease

- Smoking
- Diabetes mellitus
- Hyperlipidaemia
- Hypertension
- Male sex
- Family history of cardiac disease

Thorough assessment of the cardiovascular and respiratory systems is particularly important in patients undergoing surgery. Ischaemic heart disease (myocardial infarction, heart failure, angina), hypertension, asthma, chronic obstructive airways disease and chest infections all significantly increase the risks of anaesthesia. Where non-urgent surgery is planned, deferral until the patient's condition has improved may be necessary.

Myocardial infarction within the preceding 6 months is a significant risk factor for further infarction and peri-operative death. When possible, surgery should be postponed until after this period, and some authorities suggest a minimum of 1 year. Patients with a past history of rheumatic fever are predisposed to valvular heart disease, which can lead to heart failure and infection of the valves (infective endocarditis). Intra-oral procedures, especially those involving the teeth or gums (e.g. removal of wisdom teeth), are well recognized as risk factors for this complication. Ideally these patients should be seen by a cardiologist, who can assess cardiac function and advise about any risks of endocarditis. Patients at risk may require antibiotic cover, depending on the surgical procedure involved. Similarly, some types of congenital heart disease and all patients with artificial heart valves will require appropriate antibiotic cover (ABC) given just before surgery. Appropriate antibiotics are suggested in the British National Formulary (BNF), or alternatively the options can be discussed with a clinical micro-biologist.

The electrocardiogram (ECG) can detect previous/recent infarcts, heart strain and abnormal rhythms. Many other abnormalities may be detected, although staff need to be skilled in ECG interpretation. Further investigations are usually requested following consultation with a cardiologist. For further information the reader is referred to any standard medical text.

Chronic obstructive airways disease predisposes to post-operative chest infections and hypoxia. For elective procedures, cessation of smoking, pre-operative physiotherapy and surgery carried out in the summer months will all significantly improve post-operative recovery (Box 1.5).

BOX 1.5 Pre-operative measures to reduce post-operative chest infection

- Being aware of high-risk patients
- Banning smoking for *at least* a few days before surgery
- Timing elective surgery for the summer months
- Improving lung function in asthmatics with nebulized bronchodilators and steroids pre-operatively
- Physiotherapy
- Reserving beds on the ICU/HDU for patients who are at particularly high risk

Smokers are also at risk of lung cancer, and an increasing number of patients with oral cancer are now surviving long enough to develop lung metastases. Tuberculosis (TB) is more common than is often believed, even in developed countries. It is seen especially among the homeless and in deprived inner-city areas where poverty and overcrowding are common.

Special investigations for assessing the respiratory system are grouped under the term 'lung function tests'. These can determine the severity of chest disease and the effects of treatment. If necessary, deterioration following surgery can be monitored by serial tests. Many of the tests can be simply performed on the ward. Examples of lung function tests include the following:

- measurement of peak expiratory flow;
- spirometry to record forced expiratory volume in 1 s;
- flow–volume curves;
- airways resistance;
- specific conductance;
- arterial blood gases and pulse oximetry.

Pre-operative arterial blood gases and haemoglobin saturation (pulse oximetry) provide useful baselines against which post-operative values can be compared. The chest X-ray is of limited usefulness, but can suggest the presence of heart failure, infection or metastases. Local protocols vary, but chest X-rays may be of use in the following patients:

- those over 60 years of age;
- those with acute respiratory symptoms;
- those with oral cancer (? metastasis);
- smokers (? primary lung cancer);
- those known to have cardiorespiratory disease, but who have not had a chest X-ray within the last 12 months;
- recent immigrants who have not had a chest X-ray within the last 12 months (?TB).

However, a normal-looking chest X-ray does not exclude the presence of disease (e.g. asthma).

Diabetes mellitus

Post-operative complications are more common in diabetic patients. This is partly due to controllable factors such as blood glucose, but it is also due to unavoidable complications such as ischaemic heart disease and infection, both of which are more common in these patients.

BOX 1.6   Risks associated with surgery in diabetic patients

- Acute hypoglycaemia
- Ketoacidosis
- Ischaemic heart disease
- Hypertension (renal disease)
- Increased risk of infections (chest, urinary, wound, 'miniplates'– see trauma chapter)
- Predisposition to pressure sores

The problems that are encountered in diabetic patients undergoing major surgery are related to the period of starvation (nil by mouth) and the metabolic effects secondary to the stress of surgery itself. The brain's main source of nutrition is glucose, yet persistently high blood sugar levels predispose to infections, poor wound healing and ketoacidosis. The aim of management is therefore to minimize gross variations in blood sugar level by ensuring an adequate glucose, calorie and insulin intake. Blood glucose needs to be within normal limits pre-operatively and maintained until normal feeding is resumed following surgery. For some patients, normal feeding after surgery may be delayed for many days, especially following major resections for head and neck cancer. Pre-operative blood glucose control can be determined by urine analysis or a random blood sugar test. Blood urea and electrolyte concentrations should also be checked in order to exclude renal disaese. Pre-operatively, it is important to determine the following:

- the type of diabetes;
- the adequacy of blood glucose control;
- the treatment regime (diet, oral hypoglycaemic agent or insulin);
- established complications (e.g. cardiovascular, renal);
- the likely delay in resumption of oral feeding.

Many regimes exist for stabilizing diabetic patients in the pre-operative period (see Box 1.7)

BOX 1.7   General principles of diabetic management

- Establish good control of blood sugar long before surgery is planned
- Avoid long-acting insulin preparations or oral hypoglycaemic agents 12–24 h pre-operatively, to prevent hypoglycaemia
- Regularly monitor blood sugar
- Fast from midnight (if on morning list)
- Place the patient first on the list
- Control blood sugar levels on the day of surgery using intravenous short-acting insulin and intravenous dextrose (many regimes exist)
- Check potassium levels and supplement if necessary
- Post-operatively, make continued use of a sliding scale until an oral diet is re-established, and then restart normal regime

Sliding scales involve the continuous infusion (intravenously or subcutaneously) of short-acting insulin, using a syringe pump. The rate of infusion varies according to the patient's blood glucose, which is checked regularly (e.g. hourly, depending on its stability). The higher the blood glucose concentration, the more insulin is given. In this way hyperglycaemia can be controlled without risking profound hypoglycaemia. Sliding scales should be reviewed constantly and adjusted to achieve a relatively steady infusion rate. The aim is to establish a steady blood glucose level rather than constantly oscillating below a low and high insulin infusion rate.

In acute cases blood glucose is often grossly abnormal, usually secondary to infection, trauma or reduced oral intake. Patients are often hyperglycaemic, which can lead to diuresis, dehydration and ketoacidosis. These patients require intravenous rehydration, correction of electrolytes and infusion of short-acting soluble insulin. Regular monitoring of blood glucose, sodium, potassium and acid–base balance is essential. When rehydration is under way and some correction of acidosis and hyperglycaemia has been achieved, emergency surgery may then be carried out, continuing management during and after surgery.

Bleeding disorders

The presence of blood dyscrasias and other causes of prolonged clotting must be considered, especially when there is prolonged bleeding following minor oral surgery. Common problems include haemophilia A, haemophilia B, Von Willebrand's disease, liver disease and patients on anticoagulants. Patients with known or suspected bleeding problems need to be fully assessed by an appropriate specialist, ideally in the out-patient clinic prior to admission. With appropriate prophylactic measures (e.g. local measures, tranexamic acid, DDAVP, factor replacement or adjustment of warfarin doses) surgery can be safely carried out, although the patient may need overnight admission. Patients on warfarin need careful assessment as they may require adjustment of the dose until the INR is at an acceptable level. Opinions vary considerably with regard to what is 'acceptable', as reducing the dose of warfarin in itself is not without risks to the patient (inducing a hyperthrombotic state). However, most maxillofacial units will have established guidelines, which should therefore be adhered to closely.

Thyroid surgery

Patients undergoing thyroid surgery for hyperthyroidism must be clinically and biochemically euthyroid before surgery is undertaken. Close co-operation with an endocrinologist is essential to optimize thyroid function prior to surgery.

Nutritional assessment

'Nutritional support is an essential component of the holistic care of the patient. If neglected it has many adverse effects on the individual, decreasing the wound tensile strength, prolonging recovery, increasing susceptibility to complications and increasing the risk of mortality'(Wallace, 1994).

It is now known that one of the most important factors in wound healing is nutrition. Poor nutrition can delay healing and result in a weak, poor-quality scar and/or wounds that fail to heal. Muscle wasting prevents early mobilization and, if severe, can interfere with respiratory function, predisposing to chest infections. In addition, the immune system is also affected by malnutrition, and malnourished patients are at risk of post-operative infections, not only in wounds but also in the chest and urinary tract.

Patients may be malnourished at the time of their admission, or they may become so during their stay. This must be anticipated, especially in individuals undergoing major head and neck surgery, who may be unable to eat a normal diet for several days afterwards. In such cases nutritional support is important.

Complications of malnutrition

These include the following:

- poor wound healing;
- risk of infections;
- pressure sores;
- compromised respiratory function;
- poor mobilization
- increased recovery time;
- prolonged hospital stay.

Weight loss in cancer (cachexia) is poorly understood, but the evidence suggests that tumours and other cells release 'cytokines' (e.g. tumour necrosis factor) which have widespread disruptive effects on the body's metabolism. Patients are often also anorexic, and from a maxillofacial viewpoint reduced oral intake is greatly impaired when the cancer involves the mouth or pharynx.

BOX 1.8 Causes of malnutrition in maxillofacial surgery

- Increased requirements (sepsis, major surgery)
- Decreased intake (dysphagia, painful mouth, facial trauma, head injuries)
- Enforced starvation (prolonged nil by mouth)
- Cancer cachexia
- Nausea, diarrhoea
- Difficulty with feeding with no one available to provide enough assistance
- Unappetizing food
- Poverty and self-neglect (e.g. alcohol abuse)

Patients undergoing major head and neck surgery are particularly at risk of malnutrition from reduced oral intake. However, improved surgical techniques (e.g. internal fixation of fractures which avoids prolonged periods of intermaxillary fixation; see Chapter 11 on maxillofacial trauma) and effective pain relief now mean that most patients can at least swallow liquids soon after surgery and malnutrition is unlikely. Patients considered to be most at risk are those with advanced head and neck cancer (particularly oropharyngeal) or those obtunded in some way (e.g. head injury). All patients with established malnutrition or who are considered to be at risk following surgery should be assessed pre-operatively by a speech and language therapist and dietitian (see Chapter 7 on speech and language therapy).

Nutrients

Nutrients have been described as substances necessary for normal body function. They are found in food, but not all foods contain nutrients. Nutrients which are essential for wound healing are proteins, carbohydrates, fats, vitamin A, vitamins of the B complex, vitamin C and minerals, e.g. zinc, manganese, copper and magnesium. Proteins are the basic cellular components of all living organisms and are essential for immunity and wound healing (see Chapter 4 on wound healing). Protein depletion can prolong the inflammatory phase of wound healing, which can lead to delayed healing. Carbohydrates provide the energy for leucocyte and fibroblast function. Fats are essential for the formation of new cells and provide cellular energy. Vitamin C is essential for collagen synthesis and the inflammatory response. A lack of vitamin C can delay wound healing and result in a weak scar. Vitamin A helps to maintain the body defence mechanisms and can reduce the risk of infection. It enhances epithelialization and increases collagen synthesis. Vitamin B improves the cross-linking of collagen, and is essential for the strength and integrity of wounds. Minerals such as manganese, copper and magnesium play a role in the synthesis of collagen, and zinc helps to increase cell proliferation and epithelialization and improves the strength of collagen.

It is therefore important to remember that malnourishment is not just depletion of protein, fat and carbohydrate. Electrolytes, trace elements and vitamins must also be considered. These play vital although poorly understood roles in body metabolism, immunity and wound healing. Many tests have been suggested as sensitive indices for assessing nutritional status. However, a thorough clinical examination will often identify those patients who are most likely to be malnourished (Box 1.9)

BOX 1.9 Clinical indications of malnourishment

- Weight loss (10 per cent = mild, 30 per cent = severe)
- Apathy
- Loose skin
- Wiry brittle hair
- Sunken eyes
- Sores at the corner of the mouth
- Reduced tissue turgor
- Weak grip
- Reduced arm circumference (muscle mass)
- Reduced skinfold thickness (fat thickness)
- Pressure sores

BOX 1.10 Investigations of malnourishment

Mild
- Full blood count and film
- Serum folate
- Prothrombin time
- Serum urea and electrolytes
- Liver function tests
- Serum albumin and pre-albumin
- Plasma transferin
- Retinal binding protein

Moderate to severe
- Magnesium
- Calcium
- Phosphate
- Zinc
- Molybdenum
- Selenium
- Chromium
- Manganese

Risk factors in malnutrition

Many factors result in malnutrition, such as poverty, age, alcoholism, drug dependency, bowel disease, depression and cancer. Smoking reduces the appetite. These factors must be identified. The Royal College of Nursing (1996) states that 'nurses have traditionally played a key role in meeting the nutritional needs of the hospitalised patient'. The Royal College of Nursing have set guidelines for the role of the nurse in the nutritional support of patients. These are that the patient's nutritional needs are met, and any food preferences are identified and adhered to (e.g. vegetarian diet and any foods that relate to a patient's ethnic background or religious beliefs). If patients are unable to feed themselves they are fed in a dignified manner. Any dental problems, such as poor-fitting dentures and painful mouth conditions, are identified and treated or a more appropriate diet is provided. It is the nurse's responsibility to monitor the patient's appetite and what they are actually eating so that malnutrition does not occur. The United Kingdom Central Council (1997) stated that 'the feeding of patients and clients is not a routine task. It provides the opportunity to observe and monitor aspects of the patient's progress both psychologically and physically. Without this involvement, judgements about a patient will be made with incomplete information'.

The King's Fund (1992) states that 'up to 50 per cent of surgical patients and 44 per cent of medical patients are malnourished on admission to hospital'. It is also known that patients can become more malnourished the longer their hospitalization. On their admission to hospital the nurse should assess every patient, and those who are at risk of malnutrition or who are already malnourished should be referred to the dietitian, who will set up feeding or supplement regimes that are specifically devised for that particular patient. It is the nurse's role to ensure that these regimes are implemented and to report any side-effects or changes in the patient's condition so that the regimes can be altered according to the patient's needs.

For patients undergoing major head and neck surgery, or following major facial trauma, feeding is the major problem. They need to maintain good nutritional support to match their body's increased requirements. Patients are often fed by enteral feeding or, rarely, by parenteral nutrition. However, as soon as possible they go on to a soft or liquidized diet. The speech therapist is often needed to help the patient to learn how to masticate and swallow again. This can be a very frustrating time for patients who have to learn a task that has been very much taken for granted since childhood.

Nutritional support

This can be provided in several ways (see Box 1.11).

BOX 1.11   Sources of nutritional support

- Dietary advice/supplementation
- Nasogastric tube
- Percutaneous endoscopic gastrostomy (PEG)
- Feeding gastrostomy
- Feeding jejunostomy
- Parenteral (rare)

Not all patients require support, but the advice of a dietitian is essential, particularly for all major cases.

Dietary supplementation

'For the majority of people the general appearance of a meal is important and influences whether or not a person will eat it. People who are unwell often experience a loss of appetite, so the appearance of meals takes on a greater significance' (Cortis, 1997). When a liquidized meal is necessary, it is better to show the patient the meal before it is liquidized, so that they know what they are eating. Instead of liquidizing it all together it may be better to present the portions separately, so that again the patient can visualize what they are eating. The patient should always be treated as an individual, their needs should be assessed and, where possible, their nutritional needs and requirements should be discussed with them.

Nasogastric feeding

Complications of nasogastric feeding include nausea, vomiting, diarrhoea, hyperglycaemia, aspiration, tube misplacement and oesophageal erosions. Nausea, abdominal pain and diarrhoea may be reduced by continuous feeding with regular breaks, rather than bolus feeds. Diluted 'starter' regimes are sometimes used, depending on local practice. Diarrhoea may be due to antibiotic treatment, and can be relieved by stopping the antibiotic or by giving loperamide or codeine phosphate. The infusion may have to be slowed down temporarily.

Aspiration of the feed and misplacement of the tube can be avoided by aspirating acidic gastric contents, or by injecting air down the tube and listening to the stomach with a stethoscope. If in doubt, a chest X-ray should be taken.

Proprietary feeds may be preferred to those made by liquidizing food because their composition is known, and they are sterilized and more convenient to use. A bewildering choice of feeds is now available, although only a few are required to meet the needs of most patients. Nearly all feeds contain enough vitamins, trace elements and essential fatty acids for short-term use (less than 4 weeks), and are mostly gluten and lactose free. Patients who need feeding for more than 4 weeks will need supplementary vitamins and trace elements.

Percutaneous endoscopic gastrostomy (PEG)

This has revolutionized nutritional support following head and neck surgery. Using endoscopic techniques, a small feeding tube is placed directly into the stomach through the abdominal wall, thereby bypassing the mouth, pharynx and oesophagus. This can be done under topical anaesthesia and sedation if necessary, and is a relatively quick procedure. Feeding can be resumed the following day. In this way long-term nutritional support can be ensured and the patient is free from the discomfort of nasogastric tubes. When it is no longer needed the PEG is simply removed and the stoma closes spontaneously. Contraindications to PEG feeding include previous abdominal surgery, gross obesity, peptic ulcer, liver disease, cirrhosis and bleeding disorders.

Nutritional requirements

Most patients can be adequately nourished with 2000–2500 kcal and 17–14 g of nitrogen per day. Even catabolic patients (sepsis) rarely need more than 2500 kcal. Too high a calorie intake (e.g. 4000 kcal per 24 h) can lead to fatty infiltration of the liver. Approximate energy contents are as follows:

- glucose – 4 kcal per gram;
- fat – 10 kcal per gram.

To convert kcal to kJ, simply multiply by 4.2.

Fluid diets can meet all of the necessary requirements. Patients with impaired swallowing sometimes find a semi-solid diet easier to deal with. Commercially prepared standard feeds normally contain 1 kcal per ml and 4–6 g of protein per 100 ml. Most people's requirements are met in 2 l per 24 h. However, specialist advice from a dietitian is essential. Nausea and vomiting are less of a problem if the feed is given continuously via a pump.

Deep vein thrombosis (DVT)

Deep vein thrombosis (DVT) (venous thromboembolism) is generally uncommon following head and neck surgery. However, it is a potentially life-threatening condition (pulmonary embolism, PE), and predisposes to varicose veins, leg swelling, ulceration and skin damage. It is also *preventable*. Diagnosis is often difficult, and it has been estimated that around 50 per cent of patients with extensive thrombosis have no clinical findings. Such 'silent' thrombi are of particular concern because the condition may remain unrecognized until the patient collapses. It is therefore important that patients are assessed for risk factors and appropriate preventive measures are taken.

BOX 1.12   Risk factors for DVT

High risk
- Previous history of DVT or pulmonary embolism
- Age
- Myocardial infarction
- Obesity
- Extensive trauma
- Infection
- Congestive heart failure
- Malignancy
- Pregnancy and the puerperium
- Varicose veins
- Diabetes mellitus
- Length and type of operation
- Prolonged immobilization

Other risk factors
- Oral contraceptives
- Smoking
- Sex
- Race
- Occupation
- Type of anaesthetic
- Drugs

DVT prophylaxis

Currently, prevention is directed towards elimination of stasis in the veins, or reducing the tendency to clot in the patient. Measures include the following:

- 'TED' anti-embolism stockings;
- heparin;
- intermittent pneumatic calf compression;
- low-voltage electrical calf stimulation;
- early mobilization;
- physiotherapy;
- other prophylactic measures, including intravenous low-molecular-weight dextrans and oral warfarin.

Heparin is currently available as 'fractionated heparin' and 'low-molecular-weight' heparin, which are reported to be more effective but are also more expensive. Low-dose subcutaneous heparin (5000 units bd or tds) has been shown to reduce the incidence of DVT significantly in general surgical and orthopaedic patients. Low-molecular-weight heparins may be given once daily, which is more convenient for both staff and patient.

Steroids in surgery

Steroid cover

Patients on long-term or high-dose steroids, for whatever reason (e.g. asthma, rheumatoid arthritis, inflammatory bowel disease), are at risk of adrenocortical suppression. Following surgery, trauma and infections they are unable to mount a normal 'stress response' which can lead to metabolic disturbances and occasionally to collapse. Steroid supplementation may be required in the peri-operative period commencing on induction of anaesthesia and continued post-operatively with a reducing dose. For an 'average' nil by mouth (NBM) patient one regime might be as follows:

- major surgery – hydrocortisone 100 mg IM or IV with the premedication and then qds for 3 days, after which return to previous medication;
- minor surgery – prepare as for major surgery, except that hydrocortisone is given for only 24 h.

However, not all patients who are on steroids require supplementation, and protocols vary depending on the patient and the procedure.

Stress ulceration

This occurs in patients after prolonged physiological stresses, and is classically seen following extensive burns, major trauma and multi-organ failure. Patients undergoing surgery for head and neck cancer may similarly be 'stressed' post-operatively, particularly if their recovery is complicated. This can result in fatal gastrointestinal haemorrhage, and in such patients prophylaxis is necessary. Current measures include H_2-receptor blockade and Sucralfate.

Surgery in the elderly

Surgery and anaesthesia in the elderly patient are both particularly challenging. Although the principles of assessment in the elderly are no different to those in younger patients, some specific points are worth highlighting.

- Chronological age *per se* is no indication of risk, and careful assessment is still necessary. Contrary to general belief, most elderly people are fit. A more reliable indication is the 'biological age', i.e. how old the patient looks.
- Hypertension, ischaemic heart disease and congestive cardiac failure are all common and often undiagnosed.
- Multiple problems may coexist, not all of which are related to the current diagnosis.
- Patients are often on multiple medications. These should generally be continued throughout the peri-operative period. The potential for drug interactions must always be considered during anaesthesia or drug-prescribing. Many interactions exist, particularly when prescribing antibiotics or analgesics.
- Impaired metabolism and excretion of drugs may require lower doses.
- One problem (e.g. poor mobility) may have several causes, each of which requires attention.
- Complications are relatively common and may present non-specifically, with absence of typical symptoms (e.g. myocardial infarction without chest pain, or a urinary tract infection without dysuria). Rapid deterioration can occur if these are not recognized and treated.
- Incontinence, instability, immobility, hypothermia and confusion are common problems in the elderly. However, they may be early symptoms of underlying treatable disease, e.g. urinary tract infection (UTI).
- More time is required for recovery.
- Many elderly people live alone, and their social circumstances need to be evaluated. Early involvement of social services may prevent delayed discharge in patients who go on to become 'social' admissions.

Special points in history

- Assess disability.
- Obtain home details (stairs, access to toilet, whether alarm can be raised).
- Assess understanding and compliance.
- Social support (regular visitors, family and friends).
- The need for further care (what services are involved, home help, meals on wheels, district nurse).

More operations are now being carried out on elderly patients. This is partly because the number of elderly patients in the population is growing, but also because previously difficult procedures are no longer so with improved surgical techniques (e.g. fixation of the edentulous mandible, and advances in reconstructive surgery following ablative surgery). Improved anaesthesia, pain relief and post-operative care also mean that previously 'inoperable' patients are more likely to survive.

For major surgery, routine pre-operative full blood count (FBC), biochemistry, blood gases and chest X-ray are useful as a baseline against which post-operative investigations can be compared. This is essential in patients with longstanding medical problems and associated biochemical abnormalities. In patients undergoing surgery for malignancy, a chest X-ray is also important to exclude metastasis. A pre-operative ECG is mandatory in all elderly patients, as asymptomatic heart disease may be detected.

Further assessment of disability and handicap can be made using the Barthel Index of Activities of Daily Living (BIA). Other professionals, such as community liaison nurses, occupational therapists, physiotherapists, speech therapists and social workers, should be involved at an early stage.

Post-operatively, elderly patients are generally highly dependent on nursing care. Repeated assessment of the cardiovascular and respiratory systems is essential, and careful charting of fluid balance is necessary, as these patients are particularly prone to overload or dehydration. Elderly patients should be mobilized as soon as possible to avoid pressure sores and other complications related to prolonged immobility (e.g. chest infection, DVT).

Facial disfigurement

The importance of body image is rated highly in our society, and is perpetuated through the media on television and in glossy magazines. We often make judgements about people on the basis of what they look like, especially those areas such as the face which are on view for all to see. This is especially true of the maxillofacial patient, whose face can be permanently disfigured by trauma or cancer. Their self-perception may be suddenly altered, making it all the more difficult for them to come to terms with their own image. This is also true for their loved ones, who also have to come to terms with their partner's or relative's change in image. It is therefore essential that good counselling is given to both the patient and their loved ones in order to help them to come to terms with their loss and establish a feeling of well-being and acceptance.

Chilton (1984), cited by Salter (1988), makes the following suggestion:

Body image also plays an important part in self-understanding. How a person feels about himself is basically related to how he feels about his body. The body is a most visible and material part of one's self and occupies the central part of a person's perceptions. Body image is the sum of the conscious and unconscious attitudes that the individual has towards his body. Present and past perceptions and feelings about size, function, appearance and potential are included. A person with a high level of self-esteem will tend to have a much clearer understanding of himself.

Cancers of the head and neck can be particularly disfiguring, especially following radical surgery. The level of surgery required varies from simple excision and closure for small lesions to radical excision with free tissue transfer to fill the defect. This type of surgery also leaves scars on other areas of the body used as donor sites. Even a minor procedure can have an effect on patients, as in the case of a female patient who, having had an excision of a lesion on her nose tip and repair with a full-thickness graft, said she 'would rather be dead than have that on the end of her nose'. No amount of reassurance regarding the eventual cosmesis would change her mind and she remained very distressed, even when she returned to the out-patient department several months later when the graft was hardly noticeable. She was clearly still very distressed by the appearance of the graft.

Some defects can be repaired cosmetically with local tissues. However, others, such as defects of the nose or ear cannot, and a prosthesis is often necessary. Although custom-made, they are often not available until the patient is fully healed. This leaves them without a prosthesis for some time in the interim. The patient may also have a fear of the prosthesis falling out or being noticeable at close range.

It is extremely difficult for patients to visualize what they are going to look like following surgery, so it is essential that they receive good counselling pre-operatively. This helps them to come to terms with the post-operative result, although many may still find it difficult to adjust. In the case of cancer patients, not only are they physically different, but they also fear dying of the cancer and they fear further treatment e.g. radiotherapy. It is essential for them to know that surgery is vital and possibly life-saving, as this may help them to accept the results of such surgery.

Many patients with cancer go through the grieving process on the road to recovery, and it is important that they experience each of the stages of this process. The patient's relatives may also be going through a similar experience at this time and feel excluded or isolated. They may also need to be counselled to help them to come to terms with the situation and to help them to care for and help their loved one. Following surgery the patient should be allowed to talk about their feelings and be offered all the support they need. This should be done at their own pace, as individual patients will take different lengths of time to accept themselves. The patient can then care for him- or herself and be able to deal with any reactions he or she receives from others.

Costello (1974), cited by Salter (1988), suggests that five steps are necessary when nursing patients with altered body image.

- The patient must be helped to accept the appearance of the operation site.
- He or she must touch and explore the area.
- He or she must accept the necessity of learning to care for the defect.
- He or she should develop independence and competence in daily care.
- He or she must reintegrate his or her new body image and possibly adjust to an altered life-style.

Patients may not experience these feelings until after they are discharged home. Many of them feel safe and secure in hospital and do not feel 'out of place'. However, once home they may lose that sense of security. It is therefore important that they are given emotional and practical support by their district nurse or GP. Support groups consisting of patients who have had similar experiences are also beneficial. The group can also give practical advice as well as emotional support. Not all patients want this kind of support, and referral to a trained counsellor may be necessary.

Admission

It is essential that the ward environment is friendly and warm and that the patients and their relatives are made to feel welcome. The nurse should always speak and explain things to them at a level that they will understand, and encourage them to ask questions or voice their anxieties. In this way the nurse can build confidence in the patient that his or her needs are going to be met. It is also important for the patient to feel in control and, wherever possible, they should be involved in their own care. Responsibility should be passed back to the patient as soon as possible so that they can regain control of their life. The Royal College of Anaesthetists (1990), cited by Caunt (1992), stated that: 'it is recognised that nurses have a unique value within the health care team, as they are in twenty-four-hour contact with the patient and thus are well equipped to be aware of the physiological and psychological changes, and to develop a good rapport and ongoing verbal communication with the patient'. Therefore the nurse is in a unique position to assess the patient and their relatives and to build up a positive relationship with them. The nurse is in the best position to alleviate the fears and anxieties of the patient and his or her family.

Common fears experienced by patients include the following:

- fear of the unexpected;
- loss of self-control and independence;
- fear of pain;
- fear of the anaesthetic;
- fear of disfigurement;
- concern about whether they will be able to return to work and lead a normal life.

The patient should be correctly measured for anti-embolism stockings and taught active leg exercises. They should also be assessed for the risks of developing pressure sores, i.e. Waterlow score, and steps taken to minimize these (a pressure-relieving mattress or bed). Further assessment is usually based on a model of care, of which many exist. The most commonly used model is that of Roper, Logan and Tierney. This is divided into Activities of Daily Living which cover all of the essential needs of the patient. Assessment is an ongoing process and is not just carried out on admission. Constant reassessment, planning and evaluation of care are essential if the patient's physiological and psychological needs are to be met.

The Activities of Daily Living are as follows:

- maintaining a safe environment;
- communicating;
- breathing;
- eating and drinking;
- personal cleansing and dressing;
- eliminating;
- controlling body temperature;
- mobilizing;
- expressing sexuality;
- sleeping;
- dying.

When assessing patients it is important to determine what the patient already knows and what they have been told. This can be a way of both building on their knowledge and rectifying any misinformation. They may well have had previous surgery, and this can be helpful if the experience was a positive one.

Providing information

It is essential to inform the patient about every aspect of their care pre- and post-operatively, including the following:

- pre-operative procedures and tests, and why they are performed;
- why and when they are to starve pre-operatively;
- which type of anaesthetic they will receive and why;
- what type of wound, if any, they will have, how much scarring there will be, and in what ways this can be minimized;
- the risks of infection, how this can affect their surgery, and the precautions used to prevent such infection, e.g. prophylactic antibiotics;
- whether drains are going to be used or are likely to be, why they are used and for how long;
- whether free tissue transfer or skin grafts are required, what they are, from which part of the body they are taken, and the care required to maintain them, e.g. flap observations, fluid balance, etc;
- whether a tracheostomy is required, what care will be needed, e.g. suctioning, humidified oxygen therapy, and for how long. For permanent tracheostomies patients will need to know how to care for these themselves. It is particularly important that patients know that they will be unable to speak, but they should be reassured that the staff and their own relatives will still be able to communicate with them;
- the complications of decreased mobility, e.g. DVT, chest infection, UTI and development of pressure sores.

It may be necessary to repeat the information more than once, as patients often do not fully understand or absorb what they have been told the first time. They should be encouraged to ask questions at any stage, and this should be continually emphasized. Opportunity for this should be made available right up to the time of theatre. It has been suggested that it is 'the immediate preoperative period in which the patient receives minimal care and is most vulnerable'. Because patients are often overloaded with information during the initial admission period, if time allows it may be better practice to spread this out throughout the pre-operative period.

Discharge home

Effective discharge planning *should be commenced on admission* and involves the multidisciplinary team. It is the admitting or named nurse's role to commence discharge planning when assessing the patient on arrival. Certain aspects of community care may require some time to set in place and must therefore be anticipated. In some cases it is difficult to predict the date of discharge, but an expected date can be noted. For the same reason, early referral to the other members of the multidisciplinary team should be made, i.e. to the physiotherapist, occupational therapist, social worker, etc. Each Trust has its own discharge policy, but the main principles are the same.

Most patients who have had major head and neck surgery will require a complex discharge package, and the community services should be informed early on about what type of care and equipment the patient will need, e.g. suction machine or feeding pump. A full social history is required, including an accurate address and whether it will be suitable for the patient's needs once they have been discharged. Will there be a carer to look after them and, if so, are they physically and mentally fit to do so? For instance, an elderly wife may not be able to cope with her husband's care and he may need more specialized care or more input from social services.

The patient should also undergo a thorough assessment of how well they can carry out the activities of daily living as previously stated. For example, can they wash and dress themselves? Can they feed themselves or manage a feeding pump? This assessment is usually carried out by the occupational therapist, and in some cases a home visit with the patient is arranged to assess how well the patient can cope in their own home. Some patients may require their homes to be fitted with safety equipment such as rails. The patient's bed may need to be moved downstairs and a commode ordered. However, it is important that the relatives are kept advised at every stage of planning in order to ascertain their concerns.

The patient and their carer or carers should be taught the necessary skills for caring for the patient once they are home, e.g. tracheostomy or PEG care, removal and cleaning of obturators and prostheses, or care of grafts or flaps. They should be given adequate time to practise and become confident in the skills and techniques, and this should be supported with up-to-date and accurate information leaflets, as well as 24-hour contact telephone numbers for use in the event of a problem.

Transport should be arranged if necessary, as well as ensuring that there will be someone to greet the patient or that there is a key so that they can gain access to their home. If the patient lives alone it may be necessary for social services to arrange for the heating, etc., to be switched on and to ensure that there is food in the home when the patient arrives. The patient should be given any medications required, and a full explanation should be given to ensure that they are taken correctly and at the right times. If the patient requires dressings, an adequate supply should be sent home with them to enable the district nurse to change them. Ideally they should be dressings that are available on prescription, which is not the case for all dressings.

Finally, it is important to arrange out-patient appointments and transport for these. On discharge patients are vulnerable, as they are leaving the safety of the hospital. It is therefore essential that discharge is properly planned and that patients and their relatives are well informed. This will considerably ease any fears or anxieties.

Local anaesthesia and sedation

Sharon Maddix and Michael Perry

Local anaesthesia (LA)
Sedation

The ability to produce effective local anaesthesia (LA) in the head and neck, including the oral cavity, is an essential skill in which all head and neck surgeons should be accomplished. When necessary, local anaesthesia may be supplemented with sedation, which may be administered orally, intra-venously or by inhalation. This is particularly useful in anxious patients and in children, although it must be appreciated that sedation by itself is not a substitute for good local anaesthestic technique. With patience and a good technique, anaesthesia almost anywhere in the face, neck, scalp and oral cavity can be obtained. 'Nerve blocks' placed at key areas where large nerve trunks emerge into accessible sites (e.g. inferior alveolar nerve, infra-orbital nerve, trigeminal ganglion) reduce the volume of LA required, so large areas can be anaesthetized without overdosage. Many simple procedures are often carried out in this way (e.g. intra-oral or extra-oral biopsy, scar revision, extraction of teeth, dento-alveolar surgery), although more complex proce-dures can also be undertaken (e.g. plating of mandibular fractures, Gillies lift for fractured zygoma, eminectomy, and correction of bat ears). The potential effectiveness of this technique is demonstrated in reported cases of neck dissections and parotid surgery carried out under LA!

Local anaesthesia (LA)

Case selection is especially important when considering the suitability of a patient for surgery under local anaesthesia. Children may be extremely unco-operative, and it is inadvisable to attempt local anaesthesia by forcibly restraining the child in case of accidental injury. Similarly, confused or psychiatrically unwell patients may also be difficult to anaesthetize effectively. Surprisingly, however, there are many instances where, with careful explanation, patience and gentle technique, local anaesthesia can be obtained in those patients in whom it was originally considered unlikely.

Surgery under local anaesthesia carries a number of significant advantages for the patient, surgeon and unit alike.

- Minor treatment or investigations can be offered there and then.
- It avoids admission for general anaesthesia.
- Patients may be dealt with more quickly and discharged much earlier.
- The risks and side-effects of general anaesthesia are avoided.
- It is more cost-effective than admission and general anaesthesia.
- Many patients prefer local anaesthesia to general anaesthesia.

Local anaesthesia is also very useful in the diagnosis of facial pain. Nerve blocks (inferior alveolar, infra-orbital, supra-orbital and supratrochlear) can be used as a diagnostic test for trigeminal neuralgia or other causes of facial pain thought to be primarily due to nerve irritation (e.g. neuroma). Similarly, infiltrating local anaesthetic around the periodontal ligament of an isolated tooth with resultant pain relief strongly suggests that the tooth is the origin of the pain.

Local anaesthetic techniques

Local infiltrations and regional nerve blocks are the means by which anaesthesia is obtained. Commonly used techniques include the following.

- *Inferior alveolar (inferior dental) nerve block* – this is the method of choice for all mandibular teeth, although the more anterior ones are usually supplemented by local infiltration. Local anaesthesia is placed around the inferior alveolar nerve as it enters the mandible approximately 1 cm above and behind the wisdom tooth.
- *Lingual nerve block* – the lingual nerve runs in close proximity to the inferior alveolar nerve in the region of the third molar. This is often anaesthetized at the same time as the inferior alveolar nerve, producing anaesthesia to the lining of the floor of the mouth and the tongue on the same side.
- *Mental nerve block* – the mental nerve is a continuation of the inferior alveolar nerve as it leaves the mandible in the region of the first and second premolars and enters the lip. Bilateral blocks can anaesthetize the entire lower lip.
- *Nasopalatine block* – anaesthesia to the palatal aspects of the upper anterior teeth can be obtained by injecting local anaesthetic into the incisive papilla. However, this is extremely painful to administer.
- *Infra-orbital nerve block* – the infra-orbital nerve emerges through the cheekbone about 1 cm below the orbital rim. This can be infiltrated either directly through the overlying skin or by passing the needle intra-orally, which tends to be less painful.
- Other named blocks include the *trigeminal nerve block, long buccal block, supraorbital nerve block, posterior, superior alveolar nerve block* and *intraligamentary analgesia* (for individual teeth).

Complications of local anaesthesia

These include the following.

- Incorrect placement, as injection of local anaesthetic within the parotid fascia (e.g. when attempting to anaesthetize upper third molars) can result in temporary facial weakness. Although it is quite alarming, no permanent damage occurs and the patient should make a full recovery. An eye-patch may be required until normal eyelid closure returns.
- Muscle injury (e.g. medial pterygoid during inferior alveolar nerve injection) may result in painful muscle spasm (trismus). This usually resolves spontaneously.
- Adjacent vascular structures may be injured, resulting in local haematoma. This may also be seen following inferior alveolar nerve injection as the corresponding artery runs close by.
- Local anaesthetic may be injected directly into the circulation. This may lead to rapid onset of toxic symptoms, which can result in collapse and cardiorespiratory arrest. Rapid injection into tissues by itself may also lead to toxicity.
- Local anaesthetic should not be injected into inflamed or infected tissues. The hyperdynamic circulation locally may lead to rapid absorption of the anaesthetic. In addition, the acid environment associated with infection reduces the effectiveness of anaesthesia.
- Hypersensitivity-type reactions can occur with some anaesthetics.
- Needle-track infection is extremely rare.
- With regard to post-injection problems, it is important to tell the patient to avoid smoking, drinking hot liquids or biting the lip or cheek until sensation is fully returned.

Sedation

Sedation is a useful technique that is often employed as an adjunct to local anaesthesia in anxious patients, children and those undergoing more lengthy procedures. Patients quite often experience a sense of distortion or detachment, and may describe the experience as similar to being mildly drunk. Amnesia is a common side-effect and unpleasant memories of the procedure are unlikely. Patients often dream during the procedure and benzodiazepines in particular can induce sexual fantasies. It is therefore important to have a second person present during administration of and recovery from sedation. Sedation is not a substitute for effective local anaesthesia. If anaesthesia is inadequate, the patient will still experience extreme discomfort. Patients do not need to be starved prior to sedation, and any routine medication should be taken as normal. Informed consent, preferably written, is required both for sedation and for surgery.

Three main routes of administration are currently available, namely intravenously, orally and by inhalation.

Intravenous sedation

Intravenous sedation is the most effective method of supplementing local anaesthesia. It may be defined as 'the single injection of a single drug'. Although some surgeons deepen sedation by adding a second drug, often an opiate, this carries a significant risk of profound sedation with a very narrow safety margin. The use of multiple drugs should only be carried out by fully trained anaesthetists in a hospital setting. A working knowledge and skills in venous cannulation, drug administration, potential side-effects, reversal and monitoring is mandatory. Although collapse is uncommon, all of the staff involved must be proficient in cardiopulmonary resuscitation (CPR), and this proficiency must be kept up to date.

IV sedation is best avoided in those patients who:

- are on certain types of antidepressants, as their recovery might take longer;
- are pregnant (evidence of cleft lip or palate in babies);
- are breastfeeding;
- have respiratory conditions;
- have kidney or liver disease.

Both during surgery and afterwards monitoring is essential until the patient is fully alert and responsive. This includes frequent monitoring of the pulse, blood pressure and pulse oxymetry. Until the patient is fully awake it is advisable to maintain good intravenous access in the event of unexpected collapse, and resuscitation facilities must be immediately available. Equipment must be routinely maintained to ensure that it is in full working order and drugs have not reached their expiry date.

In selected cases one person can be both sedationist and operator. In such circumstances a second appropriate person should always be available to assist in times of difficulty. Here 'appropriate' means someone who has experience of sedation techniques and has been trained in cardiopulmonary resuscitation. At no time should the patient be allowed to lose consciousness during sedation.

Overdosage or sensitivity to benzodiazepines can result in profound sedation or loss of consciousness. Flumazenil, a specific reversal agent, can be given in such cases and should always be immediately available. However, the half-life of Flumazenil is shorter than that of the benzodiazepines, and any reversal will wear off, resulting in re-sedation after a short period of time. Multiple doses may therefore be required and patients must never be left unsupervised until they are fully alert.

Children may react inappropriately with paradoxical stimulation, and intravenous sedation is not recommended for those under 16 years of age.

Pre-operative instructions

- The patient should be warned that it is conscious sedation, and that they will therefore be awake and will still have to have the injection in the mouth.

- It is not a general anaesthetic, so the patient should eat beforehand.
- The patient *must* be escorted by a responsible adult, otherwise the procedure will not be carried out.
- Arrangements for transport home must be made, as the patient will not be allowed to drive a vehicle (or work machinery) for 24 h.

The patient should not return to work on the same day. Every patient must have their blood pressure recorded before the procedure starts, and a record must be kept of each patient who has IV sedation and how much was administered.

Administration

Good IV access should be established in case of unexpected problems. Sedative is injected slowly in small increments to a sedation level where the patient's anxiety is reduced. Once this is established, an armboard placed under the arm can help to prevent the patient from kinking the cannula or bruising the vein. The aim is not to render the patient unconscious, but to induce relaxation in a responsive patient who still has his or her protective reflexes.

Side-effects include the following:

- headaches;
- dizziness;
- drowsiness;
- amnesia;
- condensation of time;
- euphoria – this may last for 6–8 h after a 10-ml dose (the longest recorded episode of euphoria was 48 h).

After-care

- The patient should be observed for at least 20 min.
- Instructions should be given to both the patient and the escort on the after-care of the patient's mouth.
- It should be emphasized that for 24 h the patient should abstain from:
    driving a vehicle;
    operating machinery;
    business matters;
    walking alone near traffic.
- After 20 min the patient should be checked to see whether they understand everything, and they will then be allowed to leave if they feel that they are not drowsy.

Oral sedation

This is useful for mildly anxious patients, and can be administered at home prior to the appointment. However, gastrointestinal absorption varies from one patient to another, and the degree of sedation achieved is highly variable in depth and duration.

Two drugs are commonly used:

- *temazepam* – 1 h pre-operatively;
- *diazepam* – this can be given as a single dose 1 h pre-operatively, or in divided doses starting the night before.

Inhalational sedation – relative analgesia

This is a relatively safe form of sedation that is used in dentistry, although it plays little role in head and neck surgery. It is particularly useful for children. Nitrous oxide mixed with 30 per cent (minimum) oxygen is used. This has both sedative and analgesic effects. Equal mixtures of each (50 per cent), Entonox, can provide good pain relief without loss of consciousness. This is usually given by self-administration by means of a demand valve, and is often used during labour, for changing painful dressings and in emergency ambulances. Due to its low solubility, analgesia is rapidly attainable, and when it is no longer being administered the patient makes a quick recovery with no 'hangover' effect. Only a few contraindications exist, including upper respiratory tract infection and pre-existing vitamin B_{12} deficiency.

3 Day-case surgery

Janet Powell and Michael Perry

This chapter highlights important considerations when evaluating patients for day-case surgery and outlines the care of these patients. Procedures carried out on a day-case basis have been recorded as early as the beginning of the century. However, the concept of day-case surgery did not become popular until the 1960s in the USA and about 20 years later in the UK. Since then it has become more popular as advances in both anaesthesia and surgery have enabled increasing numbers of procedures to be undertaken safely in this way. Over the last few years day surgery in the UK has increased to over 30 per cent of elective surgery (all surgical specialties), and this figure continues to rise. The National Health Service Executive has now set a new target of 60 per cent by the year 2000.

Day-case surgery may be undertaken under general anaesthesia, regional anaesthesia or local anaesthesia.

Definitions

Day-cases, out-patient cases and out-patient procedures

BOX 3.1 Definition of a day-case

The Royal College of Surgeons (1992) has defined a surgical day-case as

'a patient who is admitted for investigation or operation on a planned non-resident basis, but who none the less requires facilities for recovery'

The key points in this definition are as follows.

- The patient is admitted with a view to discharge later that day.
- Admission and surgery are planned in advance.
- Facilities for recovery following anaesthesia and surgery (or investigation) are required.

BOX 3.2 Out-patients

Out-patient cases
These are planned minor procedures carried out under local anaesthesia *without* the need for 'facilities for recovery' (e.g. scar revision, apicectomy)

Out-patient procedures
These are procedures which are *unplanned* and carried out at short notice, usually during a routine out-patient clinic (e.g. marcaine injection for trigeminal neuralgia, urgent biopsy)

Facilities

The ideal facilities are a 'self-contained' unit or ward dedicated exclusively to day surgery. Experienced nursing staff trained in pre-operative selection and assessment of patients undergoing general anaesthesia and surgery are essential. Provision for post-operative recovery and the safe discharge of patients home with the support of an appropriate carer is also necessary.

ADVANTAGES

- The patient is given a fixed date and time for admission, often at the same time that they are placed on the waiting-list.
- Pre-operative assessment prevents most unexpected cancellations on the day of surgery.
- Admissions can be 'staggered' during the day to minimize waiting.

- The high turnover and reduced delay between cases mean that more patients can be treated on any particular list. This helps to reduce waiting-lists by 'clearing' minor cases whilst using in-patient beds for more complex ones.
- Patients spend minimal time away from home (this is particularly useful for children).
- Many patients prefer this to in-patient care.
- Economically, the effective use of resources and reduced staffing needs (e.g. no night staff) saves money.
- Day-case surgery is often suited to children.

DISADVANTAGES

- Appropriate case selection is essential. After the patient is placed on the waiting-list they may not be seen again until the day of surgery. It is therefore important that both patient and procedure are appropriate to day-case facilities.
- It may be difficult to carry out any pre-operative investigations on the day of surgery. Pre-assessment clinics are therefore needed for questionable cases.
- Patients need to be accompanied by a responsible adult, who must be prepared to look after them for 24–48 h post-operatively.
- Surgery and anaesthesia must be performed by experienced senior staff if post-operative complications are to be kept to a minimum and a high turnover maintained. This limits the opportunity for junior doctors' training in day-case surgery.
- Unexpected post-operative complications may require overnight admission, and provision must be made for this.
- Home circumstances must be such as to ensure adequate aftercare.
- Administration must be efficient.

Patient selection

Patients who are to undergo surgery under a general anaesthetic need to be assessed using medical, social, psychological and surgical criteria before placing them on the waiting-list. The surgeon in the out-patient department will initially decide if the operation is safe enough to be carried out as a day-case procedure. He or she must carry out a detailed medical history and physical examination, and needs to know which factors may make day surgery risky or inappropriate. For example, if there is a high risk of bleeding, difficulty in providing effective pain control or likely prolonged immobility, then the patient would benefit from a longer stay in hospital. Unfortunately, in most busy out-patient clinics, surgeons often do not have time to check fully all of the criteria for day surgery, and more detailed assessment is therefore needed. This is carried out in pre-assessment clinics (see below).

Medical considerations

Patients must be fit enough to be given a general anaesthetic from which there are no anticipated delays in recovery or significant risks of post-operative complications (e.g. chest infections, myocardial ischaemia, venous thrombosis). Several classifications exist describing anaesthetic risk or 'fitness for operation'. The classification introduced by the American Society of Anaesthesiologists (ASA) is now widely used to grade patients' fitness for anaesthesia:

Class I   – a normal healthy patient;
Class II   – a patient with mild to moderate systemic disease, caused by the condition to be treated surgically or by any other disease;
Class III – severe systemic disease or disturbance from any cause;
Class IV – severe systemic disorders that are already life-threatening;
Class V   – the moribund patient with little chance of survival for more than 24 h.

Generally speaking, patients who are not ASA Class I or II are considered to be unsuitable for day surgery.

BOX 3.3 Common medical conditions that preclude day-case surgery

- Angina or myocardial infarction in the last 6 months
- Hypertension, heart failure or open heart surgery
- Circulation problems, such as previous stroke
- Acute chest infections, asthma (mild asthma is acceptable), chronic obstructive airways disease (chronic bronchitis, emphysema)
- Diabetes mellitus (see below)
- Severe musculoskeletal disorders such as kyphoscoliosis, muscle-wasting disease and severe rheumatoid arthritis, particularly involving the neck or jaw. These make anaesthesia difficult and can delay recovery
- Degenerative nervous disease
- Epilepsy
- Renal failure
- Patients who are more than 20 per cent overweight
- Alcohol abuse
- Psychologically unsuitable cases
- Patients taking anticoagulants
- Patients taking steroids

Patients with the following conditions may not necessarily be excluded, but need to be assessed by an anaesthetist and may require further investigations (these are guidelines only, and acceptance criteria may vary from one unit to another):

- heart murmurs;
- blood clotting disorders;
- treated hypertension where diastolic pressure is 100;
- mild rheumatoid arthritis;
- patients taking diuretics (check urea and electrolytes);
- history of anaemia/heavy bleeding (check haemoglobin);
- patients regularly taking aspirin and/or non-steroidal anti-inflammatory drugs;
- diet-controlled diabetics whose urine is free of sugar;
- patients of Afro-Caribbean descent should have sickle test performed;
- any previous family history of serious general anaesthetic problems;
- alcohol intake over 21 units for men (1 'short' or half a pint of beer = 1 unit) or 14 units for women per week. If alcohol intake is excessive check liver function tests.

Social considerations

Home circumstances such as access to a telephone and inside-toilet facilities, heating, stairs, lift, etc., must be carefully evaluated. The person who will look after the patient following discharge should be assessed as well as the environment in which they will stay. People living alone and students in 'digs' are often not suitable, even though medically they may be very fit. A fit responsible adult carer must be available overnight and 24–48 h afterwards. It is important to take into account the age of the patient, e.g. a 75-year-old's spouse will be elderly and possibly frail, so they may be unable to manage. A young woman may have small children who require care. Suitable transport home (not public transport) is also important, as is the geography of the patient's home in relation to the day unit.

BOX 3.4 Social circumstances in which day surgery may not be appropriate

- The patient finds the idea of day-case surgery unacceptable
- There is no responsible adult available to accompany the patient home after surgery and look after them for 24–48 h post-operatively. This is necessary following either general anaesthesia or sedation, both of which can cause prolonged drowsiness following discharge
- The patient lives over an hour's drive from the unit
- At home, the patient does not have access to an indoor bathroom or telephone

---

Psychological assessment

It is important for the nurse to observe the patient's attitude to the following questions.

BOOKING FORM & GUIDELINES FOR THE SELECTION OF PATIENTS FOR DAY SURGERY

Name of Patient: _____   Date: _____

Date of Birth: _____   Hospital No: _____

Address: _____

_____   Tel. No. Home: _____

_____   Work: _____

GP: _____

Surgical Consultant: _____

Surgical Procedure: _____

Date of Operation: _____   Routine/Urgent: _____   Length: _____   LA/GA: _____

B/P: _____   Weight: _____   Height: _____

		Yes	No
1.	Is the patient ASA I or II?		
2.	**Have you excluded the obese?**		
3.	Have you excluded those with chronic respiratory or cardiovascular disease and unstable or insulin dependent diabetic?		
4.	Have you excluded patients with significant past anaesthetic problems?		
5.	Have you excluded operations taking more than 30 mins – 1 hour?		
6.	Have you excluded operations where there is a possibility of severe post-operative pain or haemorrhage?		
7.	Has the patient an escort to and from the DSU?		
8.	Has the patient post-operative care available at home for 24 hours?		
9.	Are the home circumstances satisfactory?		
10.	Is the mental attitude of the patient towards sickness and pain satisfactory?		

The answer to all of the above should be 'YES' if any Day Surgery is planned. If in doubt refer patient to DSU for Anaesthetic assessment.

11.	Has the patient been consented?		
12.	Is anaesthetic assessment required?		

If yes, arrange for blood tests and send only this form to DSU.

Signature
of Surgeon: _____

Please
Print Name: _____

2 Copies: 1. Medical Records
          1. Day Surgery Unit

MEDICAL RECORDS

Figure 3.1 Booking form and guidelines for the selection of patients for day surgery.

Will this be your first operation? If it is the patient's first operation they may be anxious and need reassurance. Enquire as to what operations they have had in the past.

Have you had a general anaesthetic before? If they have had problems previously they may not be suitable for day surgery. Explain the procedure and reassure the patient.

Do you know what operation you are having? It is important that the patient understands not only the operation but also the associated risks.

Will your family and carer cope at home looking after you? All general anaesthetic patients need a fit responsible person to look after them at home. Do they have other responsibilities?

Are you worried or concerned about anything to do with the anaesthetic, operation or recovery? The patient must be given ample time to answer and the nurse to listen to any concerns that the patient may have.

If the patient is unduly worried, or is anxious about having an operation and coping at home, or the carer feels unable to cope, then the patient should be offered in-patient care with an overnight stay.

Surgical considerations

The duration of surgery must be short enough to enable a speedy recovery from the anaesthetic. Recovery time increases with the duration of anaesthesia as the anaesthetic drugs accumulate in the patient, which prolongs their excretion. Around 1 h is considered to be the maximum length of time for a patient to be anaesthetized.

The risks of significant post-operative complications must be minimal. For example, the level of bleeding following removal of a submandibular gland is low but nevertheless potentially very serious if not drained immediately. Similarly, following reduction of a fractured zygoma, sight-threatening retrobulbar haemorrhage (see Chapter 10 on maxillofacial emergencies) may occur, usually within a few hours of surgery. This also requires immediate decompression if the patient's sight is to be saved. Both operations are relatively minor in terms of the surgery, and usually take less than 1 h to perform. However, these complications, although infrequent, are serious enough to warrant overnight observations. Clearly if a patient was at home when such a complication arose there would be undue delay prior to any treatment.

Adequate pain relief is also essential. Procedures that involve cutting and sharp dissection (e.g. scar revision, excision of skin lesions) are in general less painful than those which involve stretching, crushing and bruising of soft tissues (e.g. manipulation under anaesthesia, surgical removal of third molars). Although adequate pain relief can usually be provided by local anaesthetic techniques and analgesics, there is still much to be said for good surgical technique in minimizing post-operative discomfort.

BOX 3.5 Maxillofacial procedures that are commonly undertaken as day surgery

- Soft tissue procedures (e.g. scar revision, excision skin lesions, pinnaplasty)
- Temporomandibular joint (TMJ) arthroscopy or manipulation
- Selected trauma (e.g. simple fractures, lacerations)
- Sinus washout
- Endoscopy under anaesthetic (EUA) and pan endoscopy
- Nasal polypectomy
- Submucous diathermy of turbinates
- Excision of intra-oral lesions
- Surgical removal of third molar and other dento-alveolar procedures

Pre-operative assessment clinics

Pre-operative assessment clinics are particularly useful in cases of doubtful fitness. They enable the early identification of those patients who are unfit for surgery, they reduce last-minute cancellations on the day and they allow plenty of time for suitable replacements to be found.

Each day-surgery unit and/or ward usually has a written protocol for determining patient suitability. Only nurses who have had suitable training and experience should carry out a full assessment interview. This involves checking that the patient meets the necessary medical, psychological and social criteria. An anaesthetist should be available for the nurse to consult if he or she is concerned about the patient's medical history.

A simple but comprehensive health-status questionnaire is now used in most day-surgery units. This is completed by the patient during the assessment interview, well before the day of admission. The form is designed to give the nurse and clinicians indications, at a glance, of any potential problems. If the patient gives a positive response to any of the questions these need to be investigated by either the nurse, the anaesthetist or the patient's general practitioner.

During the assessment, baseline investigations (temperature, pulse, blood pressure and urinalysis) are carried out. Where necessary, further tests can be ordered, e.g. full blood count, urea and electrolytes, sickle cell test. An ECG should be performed on everyone over 50 years of age, and on hypertensives and diabetics. The results of these investigations can be collected in good time and early action may be taken with regard to any abnormal results. If abnormal findings (e.g. undiagnosed hypertension) are discovered, the patient's general practitioner can be informed and treatment started. Alternatively, the patient can be rescheduled as an in-patient if surgery needs to be carried out urgently.

Patients should be assessed 3–4 weeks before surgery. This should be done in the day-surgery centre where the patient can meet the staff and familiarize him- or herself with the unit/ward. Both the patient and the carer need to be aware of the preparation and recovery period following general anaesthesia and surgery. The needs of day-surgery patients differ greatly from those of in-patients, and they must have sufficient information to enable them to prepare themselves for surgery and post-operative care at home. Both written and verbal instructions and information must be given to enable the patient and carer to make the necessary arrangements, e.g. when to starve, and how long they will be away from work or unable to drive. If either of them are insufficiently prepared the patient may have their operation cancelled or have to be admitted as an emergency on the day. Patients need to be talked through the process by the nurse in order to alleviate their fears and anxieties. It is important not to use medical jargon, and to listen to what the patient says or asks.

The patient and carer need to know and understand the following:

- fasting arrangements – these vary between units, but clear fluids up to 3 h and food up to 6 h before surgery usually ensure an empty stomach;
- bathing/showering and shaving instructions – shave the site of operation on the day of surgery, do not use bath oil or talcum powder, etc.;
- whether to take their own medication before admission – some interactions may occur with the type of anaesthetic or surgery, e.g. the 'pill' can cause thrombosis;
- suitable clothing to wear;
- suitable transport home (not public transport or motor bike);
- suitable adult escort home;
- who will look after the patient following discharge;
- the approximate length of time the patient will spend in hospital before discharge home.

Guidelines for pre-operative assessments of patients who are to undergo a general anaesthetic

BOX 3.6 Suitable patients for day-case surgery

- Low anaesthetic risk (ASA I or II)
- Patients who are not grossly overweight
- No history of anaesthetic problems
- Patients living within 1 h of travelling time from the hospital
- Patients who have a fit, responsible adult to care for them for 24–48 h after surgery
- Patients with a co-operative and positive attitude
- Suitable transport home (not public transport)
- Satisfactory home circumstances (inside toilet, access to a telephone, heating, stairs, lift, etc.)
- Most children

**IT IS DANGEROUS TO DRIVE, RIDE A BICYCLE, OPERATE MACHINERY OR
USE A COOKER ON THE DAY YOU HAVE A GENERAL ANAESTHETIC**

Day: _____ AM/PM: _____ Date: _____

Name: _____

Surgical Consultant: _____

No: _____

Operation: _____

Date of Birth: _____

ADULT DAY SURGERY UNIT PRE-OPERATIVE QUESTIONNAIRE

PLEASE TICK CORRECT ANSWERS

YES NO

NURSING OBSERVATIONS:

1. Have you had anything to drink in the last 3 hours?

Pulse   bpm.

2. Have you had anything to eat in the last 6 hours?

3. Will you have to go home alone?

SpO_2

4. Will you have a fit responsible adult when you get home?

B.P.

5. Will this be your first operation?

6. Have you had any problems with anaesthetics?

ECG

6a. Post op nausea/vomiting ☐   motion sickness ☐
    pregnancy sickness ☐

BMI

7. Has any of your family had problems with anaesthetics?

Wt.   Kg.

8. Do you have a cough, cold or nose trouble?

9. Have you had any serious illnesses in the past?

Height

10. Have you had heart disease, rheumatic fever or high blood pressure?

Temp.   deg. C.

11. Do you get breathless or chest pain on exercise or at night?

L.M.P.

12. Do you get swollen ankles?

13. Do you have asthma, bronchitis or other chest diseases?

List Allergies Here:

14. Do you smoke (indicate no. per day)?

15. Have you ever had a convulsion or fit?

16. Do you have arthritis or muscle disease?

17. Do you suffer from anaemia or other blood disorders?

18. Do you bruise easily or bleed excessively?

19. Have you ever had liver disease or been jaundiced?

List Drugs Here:

20. Do you drink more than a moderate amount of alcohol?

21. Have you ever had kidney disease?

22. Do you have diabetes (sugar in the urine)?

23. Do you have any known allergies (include elastoplast)?

24. Are you currently taking any drugs or other medications?

25. Do you have any crowns, loose teeth or artificial teeth?

26. Do you wear contact lenses?

27. If female, are you pregnant?

R   L

28. Do you suffer from indigestion, reflux or heartburn?

NURSES SIGNATURE: _____   **DATE:** _____

PATIENT'S SIGNATURE: _____   **DATE:** _____

A1100/1039

Figure 3.2   Adult day surgery unit pre-operative questionnaire.

BOX 3.7 Unsuitable patients for day-case surgery

- Those who do not fulfil the above criteria
- Patients who are anxious and do not want day surgery
- Any patient who has impaired mobility and is likely to require skilled nursing care
- Operation taking longer than 1 h
- Operation where there is a risk of post-operative pain or significant haemorrhage

Patients who are unable to fulfil the social criteria may be managed as 'day-stay' cases. Here patients attend on the morning of surgery but are admitted post-operatively for 24–48 h requiring only minimal care.

Creating the right ambience

This is of prime importance. A non-clinical environment alone is not enough, but needs a group of staff with good 'people' skills. Care must be provided in an enthusiastic, friendly, cheerful way by a team of nurses trained in day-case care.

Patient information is essential. Both the surgeon and the nurse need to spend time in the clinic informing the patient about the operation, including what symptoms to expect when they get home, and who to contact in an emergency. Day-unit staff should take each patient through the pre-operative instructions, e.g. fasting, etc. The patient needs to be told what will happen on the day of surgery and what to bring with them. Printed leaflets and/or cassette recordings advising patients not to drive, return to work or use heavy machinery for 24 h are helpful although not essential. On discharge, the patient should be given a letter for their GP indicating what further treatment is required (e.g. wound dressing, suture removal). A supply of oral analgesics, anti-emetics if necessary and instructions about out-patient review should also be given to the patient.

Pain control

Effective pain relief is important when the patient is to be discharged soon after surgery, and they must not be allowed to return home if in moderate or severe pain. The choice of analgesic must have minimal side-effects such as nausea or drowsiness. Most day-surgery units have a protocol for pain management which may include the following principles.

- Pain control should be addressed on admission and before surgery begins.
- To measure patients' pain, pain-scoring systems are available such as linear analogue scales (0–10, ranging from no pain to severe pain) or a verbal rating (no pain, slight, moderate, severe pain).

- Use of long-acting, regional local anaesthesia (e.g. marcaine infiltration or nerve blocks following dento-alveolar or soft tissue surgery).
- Oral analgesics, e.g. co-proxamol, co-dydramol or paracetamol and, in selected cases, non-steroidal anti-inflammatory drugs, e.g. Voltarol. These may be given prior to surgery and post-operatively. Alternatively suppository analgesics may be given, but the patient must consent to this beforehand.
- Regular administration of analgesics to avoid break-through pain.
- Avoid opiates.

Pain audits should be carried out at regular intervals to establish that the analgesia that is being prescribed is adequate.

Post-operative nausea and vomiting

The patient's discharge will be delayed if post-operative nausea and vomiting occur. Prevention is better than treatment, and an anti-emetic given prophylactically whenever possible is far better than waiting for the patient to vomit. Certain factors affect the incidence of post-operative nausea and vomiting, and it helps if the nurse can identify those patients who are at risk and help to plan their care. Risk factors include the following:

- previous surgery – history of nausea and vomiting;
- motion sickness;
- type of surgery;
- type of anaesthetic;
- use of opiates or post-operative analgesia;
- sitting up too quickly and rapid movement after an anaesthetic;
- fasting for long periods.

Haemorrhage

This is very uncommon in day-surgery units, but must not be overlooked as this can delay or prevent the discharge of the patient. The nurse must observe the operation site at regular intervals for signs of haemorrhage. This includes monitoring the patient's pulse and blood pressure at regular intervals for early signs.

Discharge arrangements and post-operative instructions

The care of the post-operative patient is the responsibility of the ward nurses. The successful, quick discharge of patients is dependent on an uncomplicated post-operative recovery, and therefore the following must be adequately controlled:

- pain and discomfort;
- post-operative nausea and vomiting;
- bleeding/haemorrhage – no patient should be discharged if there is more than a minimal amount of bleeding or drainage.

Discharge criteria

It can be difficult to assess when a patient has fully recovered from general anaesthesia. Memory for new facts can take several hours to return to normal following brief general anaesthesia, but no single test can determine when a patient is free from the effects of anaesthetic drugs. Discharge criteria must be adhered to and agreed on by the multidisciplinary team. Usually a senior nurse or doctor determines when the patient is sufficiently recovered to be discharged safely, based on stable vital signs and whether the patient can dress, tolerate foods or fluids, walk unaided and void urine. This must be documented in the notes. If patients do not meet these criteria, a bed will have to be made available for observation of the patient overnight.

BOX 3.8   Patient 'check-list' before discharge

- The patient must be street fit for discharge after a general anaesthetic. Adequate time must be allowed (at least 2 h from the first stage of recovery) before discharge home to ensure a full uneventful recovery
- Stable vital signs
- Alert and orientated
- Tolerating oral fluids
- Able to sit unaided and walk aided
- Responsible adult escort accompanying the patient
- Written and verbal discharge instructions given
- Mobility aids provided
- Follow-up appointment
- Medications to take home
- Letter faxed to general practitioner
- District nurse
- Practice nurse
- Operation site checked
- Cannula removed
- No pain/minimal pain

Prior to discharge, written and verbal post-operative instructions should be given to reinforce those that were explained prior to surgery.

BOX 3.9 Post-operative instructions

- Explaining how pain or discomfort can be controlled by using local anaesthetic and taking analgesics regularly goes a long way towards alleviating pain once the patients gets home
- Other drugs (e.g. anti-emetics or antibiotics) – when the next dose is due and the possible side-effects and what to do about them
- What to expect and how the patient will feel (time-scale); the patient must not drive, operate machinery, use a cooker, sign contracts or drink alcohol for 24 h after a general anaesthetic
- Advice on resting, driving, drinking, eating and returning to a normal daily routine
- Arrangements for out-patient follow-up
- Who to contact in an emergency or if the patient or carer is concerned or worried
- Follow-up arrangements (e.g. removal of sutures or district nurse/practice nurse arrangements)
- Use of home facilities (e.g. toilet, stairs, heating, lift and telephone); when to bathe and shower and when to resume normal activities/return to work
- Make adequate alternative arrangements if the patient is responsible for the care of children, elderly relatives or pets

Pre-medication

To avoid post-operative drowsiness this is generally not prescribed routinely for day patients. However, very anxious patients may benefit from a short-acting oral benzodiazepine such as temazepam taken 1 h pre-operatively. In such instances the patient must not attend alone or drive to the unit.

Complications

Serious complications are rare if day-case surgery is confined to short, minor procedures in fit patients. However, minor complications include the following:

- impaired psychomotor function – this is expected after general anaesthesia and is potentially dangerous. Up to 30 per cent of patients may feel drowsy after their return home, and impairment has been found 8 h after general anaesthesia that lasted for only 10 min. Reaction times may be prolonged for up to 48 h afterwards;
- anorexia, malaise, fatigue, dizziness and headache – each of these occurs in around 10 per cent of patients after general anaesthesia and can be severe enough to disrupt normal activities for the first 24 h;
- nausea with or without vomiting – this rarely persists beyond the first post-operative day, but nausea may last for 2 days;

AFTERCARE FOR PATIENTS HAVING DENTAL
EXTRACTIONS/SURGERY – (ADULTS)

YOU MUST NOT FOR THE FIRST 24 HOURS AFTER A GENERAL
ANAESTHETIC:

1. Drive or operate machinery
2. Drink alcoholic beverages
3. Stand for long periods
4. Make any important decisions or sign contracts for up to 24 hours after
    having an anaesthetic as your concentration will be impaired and you
    may be drowsy

FOR THE REST OF THE DAY

Keep the patient quiet and relaxed at home.
NO rinsing.
Lukewarm liquids and food only.
Avoid hard foods.

The tooth socket should not be touched.

Paracetamol or similar may be given if needed.

NEXT DAY

A warm-water mouthwash may be gently used three times a day to promote
healing. Normal toothbrushing should be resumed, although care should be
taken until the tooth socket is healed.

In isolated instances bleeding may start again. If this should occur:

1. Sit patient down with head and shoulders raised.

2. A freshly laundered handkerchief should be made into a pad, placed
    over the socket and the patient asked to bite into the pad for at least 15
    minutes.

IF BLEEDING IS STILL TROUBLESOME AFTER THIS, PLEASE CONTACT:

Figure 3.3   Aftercare for adult patients having dental extractions/surgery.

- psychological problems may occur if the patient becomes conscious during
  general anaesthesia. This is very rare, but is more likely to occur during
  day-case anaesthesia because no premedication is given and the anaesthetic is kept as light as possible. Psychological treatment may be required
  and it is essential that the anaesthetist concerned is notified;
- minor trauma to the airway is common – sore throat and hoarseness can
  last up to 7 days;

- nerve injury has been reported to occur in 1 in 1000 operations, but is likely to be rarer among day-cases. This is usually due to faulty transfer of the patient to and from the operating table, but fortunately recovery is almost always complete. Severe muscle pain may occur after 24 h if suxamethonium is given to relax the vocal cords for intubation. This typically affects the shoulder and neck muscles, and seems to be more common in fit, ambulant patients;
- back pain is common after surgery, especially in patients who have previously suffered from backache or arthritis, or after long operations;
- pain at the IV injection site;
- difficulty with micturition;
- complications specific to the operation.

Emergency admissions

On occasion the patient may not meet the discharge criteria and will be unable to go home. The main reasons for this are poor pain control, nausea and vomiting, or a surgical complication. Once a decision has been made to admit the patient, the patient and their family or carer should be informed. Each day-surgery unit/ward should have a policy for admitting patients for an overnight stay.

Follow-up

Telephone follow-up service

A telephone call should be made to all patients on the following day in order to provide advice and support. Permission to telephone the patient should be obtained from them before discharge. Some patients may not have informed their families that they were going into hospital to have an operation.

A structured questionnaire should be compiled and used to obtain valuable data with regard to the following:

- pain control and any specific problems;
- post-operative nausea and vomiting;
- sore throat;
- headache;
- sleep;
- privacy;
- parking;
- bleeding/dressings;
- pre-admission information;
- community services.

This information is invaluable to the entire multidisciplinary team, and all of the data collected can be used in audits to bring about changes in practice and improve quality standards which in the long term will benefit the patients and their carers.

Community services

Good communications and regular liaison with the community staff and general practitioner are essential, as these will dispel any anxieties and keep them informed of any changes in surgical technique, anaesthetics, pain relief, dressings and after-care.

Wound healing, soft tissue trauma and scar management

4

Caroline Evans and Michael Perry

Wound healing
The closure of wounds
Wound assessment and classification
Wound cleansing
Pain and wound management
Methicillin-resistant *Staphylococcus aureus* (MRSA)
'Soft' tissue injuries of the head and neck
Skin grafts
Scars

Intact skin and mucosa prevent micro-organisms from infecting deeper structures, particularly bone. Saliva and exudates from around the gingiva (gums) contain antibodies and 'growth factors' which enable rapid wound healing and prevent infections from developing. These are essential in view of the numerous and varied bacteria that are present in the normal mouth. Elsewhere, infections may arise secondary to skin commensals (normal inhabitants of the skin), or from contact with another source (e.g. MRSA; see below).

Skin is also essential for maintaining body fluids, as is demonstrated following extensive burns where fluid loss from the exposed tissues may precipitate hypovolaemic shock. In the head and neck, unrepaired wounds may produce loss of function of important structures (e.g. eyelids), resulting in significant morbidity. In addition, poor repair and after-care may result in unacceptable scarring with distortion of the surrounding stuctures.

The head and neck have a very rich blood supply which helps to fight infection and improves healing. Following trauma, partially avulsed skin, even if it is attached by only a small pedicle, may still have a good enough blood supply to enable it to heal if replaced. The importance of a generous blood supply is highlighted in the irradiated patient, in whom wound breakdown and infection are more common following surgery or injury.

Wound closure is a most effective form of analgesia.

Wound healing

This can be divided into the following categories.

- *First intention or primary wound healing.* The wound is closed by sutures, staples or skin closure strips ('steristrips') without delay and without any intervening gaps. The wound heals within 14 days as there is very little tissue damage.
- *Secondary intention (granulation) or secondary wound healing.* The skin edges are not closed but left apart, mainly due to tissue damage and/or loss. The wound is encouraged to granulate from its base by development of connective tissue and blood vessels on its surface. This is seen in cavity wounds. The healing time is unpredictable, but can be lengthy.

Phases of wound healing

Wound healing is divided into stages which vary from one author to another. Four phases will be described here, although there is often a large degree of overlap between them.

INFLAMMATORY PHASE

Inflammation is the body's immediate response to trauma (including surgery), being a reaction to tissue damage and/or invasion of bacteria. Initial vasoconstriction occurs and a loose fibrin clot forms a 'plug' that loosely unites the skin edges. Wound strength at this stage depends on the suture, and breakdown during this period is the result of poor closure. In response to tissue damage, mast cells release histamine, resulting in vasodilation, increased capillary permeability and swelling. Neutrophils are attracted by kinins which are also important in the appreciation of pain (see Chapter 5). As the capillaries dilate, tissue fluids rich in plasma proteins, antibodies, red cells, white cells and platelets 'leak' into the tissues. Platelets release growth factors and fibronectin which promote cell migration and wound healing. Macrophages are attracted, and these remove any wound debris, thereby beginning the process of repair (Seton Healthcare, 1993). The signs of inflammation are heat, swelling, redness and pain.

RECONSTRUCTIVE PHASE

Macrophages stimulate the formation of fibroblasts which multiply, migrate along fibrin threads and produce collagen. Fibrin is produced as early as the second day and forms a haphazard framework for wound healing. Immature blood vessels begin to regrow (angiogenesis), providing oxygen and nutrients to the healing wound. The wound therefore becomes filled with capillary loops and collagen fibres known as 'granulation tissue' which appears deep red in colour and bleeds easily. Granulation tissue is abundant in secondary intention healing, although it is not seen in a wound which has been primarily closed. This phase can last up to 24 days (Seton Healthcare, 1993).

In addition, the wound undergoes contraction. This may be responsible for 40 to 80 per cent of wound closure (Irvin, 1987).

EPITHELIALIZATION OR PROLIFERATIVE PHASE

Epithelial cells at the wound edges and remaining hair follicles migrate across the surface in a leap-frogging fashion: 'each cell moves two or three cell lengths then stops with cells coming up from the rear to continue the process' (Garrett, 1997). This process can only take place over a healthy moist wound. If infection or debris are present the inflammatory phase is prolonged and migration will not take place. 'Scabs' are separated from the wound by proteolytic enzymes and the vascularity decreases. Collagen continues to be produced, resulting in a red, raised and often unsightly scar. Wound strength increases with the formation of granulation tissue and collagen, and the tensile strength increases rapidly. However, this is still relatively weak and can stretch if unprotected.

MATURATION PHASE

Vascularity of the wound continues to decrease and the scar changes colour, fading to a silvery-white appearance. The haphazardly placed collagen fibres reorganize themselves, increasing the strength of the scar and tending to lie at right angles to the wound. At 1 year, 70 per cent or more of the original tissue may be regained, but scar tissue is never as strong as unwounded tissue.

Secondary intention healing

Wounds may gape because of destruction of tissue by trauma or infection, coupled with the elastic pull of the dermis on each side. This defect initially fills with blood clot, which dries to form a scab. The scab is gradually lifted at its edges until it falls off. In larger wounds, the growth of epithelium is more easily seen. Re-epithelialization is enhanced in a moist environment, where scab formation is reduced.

The wound heals from below upwards. Capillary loops bud and fibroblasts proliferate to form granulation tissue. This gives a velvety appearance to the wound. Myofibroblasts present in the wound contract and reduce the volume of the defect. These changes are accompanied by re-epithelialization.

The difference between first intention and second intention healing is quantitative only.

Risk factors in wound breakdown

General factors include the following:

- advanced age;
- malnutrition (protein, vitamins, trace elements);
- anaemia;
- uraemia;
- jaundice;
- malignancy (cachexia);
- chronic steroid therapy;
- diabetes mellitus;
- nutritional deficiencies (vitamin C, vitamin K, hypoproteinaemia, zinc);
- chemotherapy and radiotherapy.

Local factors include the following:

- tension;
- infection;
- crushed tissues (forceps, tight sutures);
- poor tissue vascularity (e.g. after irradiation);
- foreign body (e.g. dirt, gravel, glass);
- necrotic tissue (crushed, excessive use of diathermy);
- haematoma.

Classification of wounds

Wounds may be classified as 'tidy' or 'untidy' (see Box 4.1). Tidy wounds have the greatest chance of healing with minimal scar formation.

BOX 4.1   Classification of wounds

Tidy wounds
- Sharp incision
- Uncontaminated
- Less than 6 h old
- Low-energy trauma

Untidy wounds
- Ragged edge
- Contaminated
- More than 12 h old
- High-energy trauma
- Crushed tissue
- Burns

The closure of wounds

In a similar way to healing this may be classified as 'Primary', 'Delayed Primary' or 'Secondary'.

PRIMARY CLOSURE

'Tidy' wounds are closed as soon as possible with meticulous haemostasis and accurate repositioning of the tissues. Deep wounds are often closed 'in layers' using resorbable sutures to close the deeper tissues (e.g. deep cervical fascia). In some cases where tissue has been lost or severely damaged, trimming of the edges may convert an untidy wound to a tidy one which can then be closed primarily. However, compared to the rest of the body trimming is usually kept to a minimum. If doubt exists about the viability, tissue is often left. To excise tissues on the face widely may lead to difficulties in closing the defect cosmetically, particularly near the eyes, nose and mouth, which may become distorted. There should be no tension across the wound. In cases where tension exists as a result of tissue loss, undermining of the skin, local flap closure or skin grafts may be used.

DELAYED PRIMARY CLOSURE

When doubt exists about the status of a wound, it can be maintained with moist dressings, antiseptics and antibiotics for up to 72 h. This is useful in heavily contaminated wounds and those more than 6 h old. Dead tissue will then 'declare itself' and can be excised, allowing primary closure. Following excision of obviously necrotic tissue, a non-adherent dressing is placed or the wound is lightly packed. It is inspected under sterile conditions after several days, and if there is no evidence of further necrosis or infection, it can then be closed.

SECONDARY CLOSURE

This is the same as secondary wound healing.

Further wound management

This may be defined as 'the pursuit of permanent, functional and aesthetic healing of a patient's wound through the promotion of physiological healing and the prevention or elimination of factors – whether local, systemic or external – that disturb healing' (International Committee on Wound Management, 1992).

To treat wounds effectively it is therefore important to have an underlying knowledge of the process of wound healing. Any break in the skin's integrity can be termed a 'wound', and this can be caused in a number of ways:

- trauma (including surgery);
- circulatory failure (e.g. leg ulcers);
- pressure on the tissues (e.g. pressure ulcers).

Bleeding with clot formation occurs in traumatic wounds, where as in pressure-related wounds there is occlusion of the local circulation, resulting in tissue necrosis. Circulatory failure results in poorly oxygenated tissues, which predisposes towards breakdown and poor healing.

The wound-healing environment

Many intrinsic and extrinsic factors, including nutrition, stress, lack of sleep, inappropriate dressing, infection, slough and necrosis, can delay wound healing, causing frustration to both the patient and their carers. It is therefore important that the wound is given the correct environment to aid healing. Turner (1982) described the features of the 'optimum dressing'. These are criteria on which nurses can base decisions about wound care products.

The 'optimum dressing' should:

- maintain high humidity at the wound/dressing interface;
- remove excess exudate;
- allow gaseous exchange;
- provide thermal insulation;
- be impermeable to bacteria;
- be free of particles and toxic wound contaminants;
- allow removal without causing trauma to the wound.

In addition to Turner's criteria it should also be comfortable for the patient whilst *in situ* and should not cause distress or pain on removal.

Topham (1994) also stated that a wound should afford the following:

- sufficient moisture to encourage healing without encouraging bacterial or fungal growth;
- protection from mechanical damage;
- favourable pH (3.5–7);
- favourable temperature;
- time to heal – minimum dressing changes;
- it should be clean.

Wounds therefore heal more effectively in a moist, warm environment, which the new-generation dressings now provide. Epithelial cells can migrate easily, decreasing the healing time. Pain from the wound is reduced as exposed nerve endings are not allowed to dry out and the body's natural autolytic response to deslough is increased.

Wounds heal at a constant warm temperature of 37°C. Research has shown that it can take a wound 40 min to regain the correct temperature and up to 3 h for normal cell activity to return following a dressing change. It is important whenever possible to reduce the number of dressing changes. Historically some dressings have been changed up to three to four times a day. This means that wound healing could potentially have been delayed by up to 12 h or more. In addition, too frequent dressing changes increase the risk of infection in the wound and the risk of cross-infection to other patients. However, a heavily exudating wound with 'strike-through' also presents a risk by providing a path for infection in both directions.

Some dressings, such as gamgee and gauze, can leave fibres in a wound and delay healing by prolonging the inflammatory phase. This can also result in hypertrophic scarring. New-generation dressings are now particle-free, so reducing this risk.

Dressing changes should be as pain-free as possible, although this is not always achievable. However, they can be made more tolerable with the use of appropriate analgesia, the correct technique of removal and application, and use of the correct type of dressing. Pain is often caused by the selection of an inappropriate dressing or the appropriate dressing being applied incorrectly.

Wound assessment and classification (see also Chapter 6)

Only since the 1930s has the treatment of wounds become the role of the nurse, and this is even more so today with the rapidly growing development of the wound-care specialist. Wound assessment is the most important area in aiding wound healing. The wound should be assessed at dressing changes and the appropriate dressing decisions then made. Cooper (1990) stated that there is an 'obvious lack of valid and reliable methods by which nurses can evaluate healing status'.

There are many methods by which to assess a wound. The most common approach is to measure the width and depth of the wound or to trace an outline to compare at the next dressing change. The most obvious way to assess a wound is by inspection. The following five groups into which wounds can be categorized will be described:

- black or necrotic;
- infected;
- sloughy;
- granulating;
- epithelializing.

Black or necrotic wounds

These are covered with a dry hard eschar which can vary in colour from off-white/yellow to brown/black or a mixture of these colours. This is caused by ischaemia of the tissues. The eschar can mask the size of the wound and may increase in size if it is not debrided. This can be achieved by surgery or chemical or biochemical means. Surgery is not always the best option for the patient, so dressings such as hydrocolloid or hydrogel or an enzymatic desloughing agent should be used. If a cavity wound is necrotic it can produce a heavy exudate and become very offensive. Alginate dressings may be appropriate for controlling the exudate.

Infected wounds

All wounds have bacteria present, but many do not show clinical evidence of infection, i.e. purulent pus (Meers, 1981) or cellulitis. Commensal organisms do not necessarily delay healing and do not necessarily cause infection. Traditional signs of infection include the following (Cutting, 1996):

- abscess formation;
- cellulitis;
- discharge;
- localized heat;
- localized pain;
- oedema;
- breakdown of the soft tissue or the epithelium;
- defective granulation tissue which is friable and easily bleeds, and discoloration of granulation tissue;
- pocketing at the base of the wound;
- delayed healing compared to that which is expected, and wound breakdown;
- abnormal smell.

A wound swab should always be taken if infection is suspected, as this will ensure that the correct antibiotics are prescribed. Antibiotics are not always required, but if they are they are often prescribed prior to the swab result. If the organism is not sensitive and the wound is not improved this should be changed once the result is known. In conjunction with antibiotics the wound can be treated topically. Flammazine is useful when *Pseudomonas* is present, and iodine-based dressings have been shown to be effective against methicillin-resistant *Staphylococcus aureus* (MRSA). Hydrocolloids and hydrogels are also useful, but not when there is excessive exudate. An alginate may be appropriate in this case, but will require changing daily.

Sloughy wounds

These consist of dead neutrophils bathed in wound exudate. The wound has a white/yellow appearance. Macrophages are able to remove the slough in the correct environment, such as is provided by a hydrocolloid or hydrogel. Sometimes there is excessive exudate. Again an alginate is appropriate for controlling this. If slough is present in a cavity, alginate ribbon or rope can be used.

Granulating wounds

These are red and granular in appearance. They bleed easily as the capillary loops are friable. Granulation tissue gradually fills the wound, so reducing its size and depth. Dressings such as hydrocolloids, hydrogels, foams and alginates are all useful in low-exudating granulating wounds, and in a more heavily exudating wound an alginate or foam dressing can be used. In a granulating cavity an alginate ribbon or rope can be used or a foam cavity dressing. Some granulating wounds develop excess granulations which are raised above the skin edges. Preparations such as silver nitrate sticks can be used to cauterize the excess. Terracortril ointment may also be used, but research into the effectiveness of this preparation is lacking. Foam dressings are also useful for reducing overgranulations.

Epitheliliazing wounds

These have pink/white tissue present as the epithelial cells spread over the granulating tissue. A moist, warm environment needs to be maintained as well as one that is protective. Dressings such as hydrocolloids and foams are therefore appropriate.

Wound cleansing

The general aim of wound cleansing is to remove any organic and inorganic debris from the wound before an appropriate dressing is applied. Persistent debris can delay the healing process or may result in infection. It is important when assessing the wound to decide whether it requires cleansing at all. Tomlinson (1987) found that instead of removing bacteria from the wound, swabbing only redistributes them. If the wound is clinically clean with no signs of infection or other matter, then it may be better not to cleanse it.

A number of antiseptics are available for cleansing wounds, but it is generally thought that they can delay healing and harm the tissues. Sterile saline solution or water are not harmful to the wound and are recommended. However, swabbing a wound can damage granulating tissue and may leave small fibres in the wound which can be a focus for infection. It is much better to *irrigate* wounds where possible, although in some areas, such as around a tracheostomy, swabbing is a much safer option. The pressure required to irrigate a wound successfully is unclear, and too high a pressure can also harm the wound, while too low a pressure will not remove any debris. Products are available on the market, such as Steripod in a squeezable vial form and Irriclens in a canister, but there is uncertainty about the amount of pressure that they exert. A 35-ml syringe and a 19-gauge needle can be used, which should not exert too much pressure on the wound. When using any solution to cleanse a wound it is important that it should be warmed prior to use. This can help to maintain the wound at body temperature.

Tap water is increasingly being used to cleanse wounds. A study by Angaras *et al.* (1992) showed that there was no difference between wounds cleaned with tap water and those cleaned with a saline solution. Certainly chronic wounds which are already colonized can be showered or bathed in tap water, e.g. when the patient is bathing, thus making it unnecessary for the wound to be cleansed afterwards. Wounds that are directly closed can be bathed 48 h afterwards. However, if skin closure tapes are used the wound must remain dry, so a waterproof film dressing can be applied prior to bathing. The problem with bathing or showering patients in the hospital setting is the risk of cross-infection, and guidelines should be followed.

For those patients who are unable to use the bath or shower, a clean bowl and warm tap water can be used, particularly to wash the extremities. Bathing and personal hygiene are important to all of us, but especially to those patients who have an offensive smelling tumour or wound. Wherever possible patients should be allowed to bath as they wish.

When choosing a method for cleansing a wound, first consider whether the wound requires cleansing. If so, which method is in the best interests of the patient and the wound? The patient's life-style and needs should always be considered, as it is not always feasible for a patient to take time off work or have someone look after their children. The wound should be constantly evaluated so that when it is clinically clean cleansing can be stopped.

Pain and wound management

For many patients wound-dressing changes are a painful experience. It is the responsibility of the nurse to ensure that dressing changes are as pain-free as possible. The correct dressing needs to be selected. For example, since dry nerve endings are painful, a hydrocolloid or hydrogel is advisable to rehydrate the tissues.

Stress and anxiety increase the level of pain, as does the feeling of loss of control. Research conducted by Hayward (1975) suggested that information given pre-operatively reduced the amount of analgesia required by the patients post-operatively. From this it is clear that a full and detailed explanation should be given to the patient prior to dressing changes. Where possible the patient should be allowed to remove their own dressing, which provides them with a sense of being in control.

Very often it is the anticipation of pain which can increase that which is actually felt, especially if the patient has already experienced pain at a previous dressing change. Pre-emptive analgesia is essential from both a physical and a psychological viewpoint. The same can be said for the self-administration of Entonox during dressing changes. This again gives the patient an element of control over the situation.

Methicillin-resistant *Staphylococcus aureus* (MRSA)

MRSA is a human pathogen that is resistant to a number of antibiotics, not only methicillin. Some strains show the potential to become epidemic (EMRSA). To most fit and healthy people MRSA is not a threat. However, it can cause serious harm to those undergoing major or even minor maxillo-facial surgery.

It is not possible at the outset to detect which strains are epidemic, so infection-control guidelines are essential to prevent cross-infection between patients. The pathogen can colonize a particular environment (e.g. nose or throat) without producing any disease, although it can also cause infection resulting in pyrexia and septicaemia. Staphylococci are Gram-positive organisms that grow on the surface of the skin, in the nostrils, mouth, umbilicus and perineal areas. Since the introduction of antibiotics, *Staphylococcus aureus* has shown a history of resistance, first to penicillin and then to methicillin in the 1960s. Vancomycin is the antibiotic most commonly used to treat patients with MRSA, but there are now concerns regarding resistance to it (VRSA).

Individuals at risk include:

- immunocompromised patients;
- the elderly and neonates;
- patients with wounds or skin lesions;
- patients who have had one or more hospital admissions in the past year;
- patients who have been transferred from other areas where MRSA is prevalent;
- patients admitted from abroad.

The principal method of cross-infection is thought to be hand carriage, although it can also be airborne. Other sources include clothing and bedding. Therefore the only way to limit the spread of the pathogen is by adhering to sound infection control policies and effective hand-washing techniques. Each Health Trust should have an infection control policy for the prevention of spread of this and any other disease. Basic principles include:

- an effective hand-washing policy;
- education of patients and their relatives in hand-washing and its importance;
- a clean and clutter-free environment with clean work surfaces;
- readily available aprons, linen and the appropriate method of disposal and waste bags;
- staff education programmes as well as good staffing levels;
- good aseptic technique when dressing patients' wounds;
- minimal movement of patients between areas and other hospitals;
- up-to-date policies and procedures for the reduction of cross-infection, as well as advice from the infection control team;

- screening of patients prior to transfer to other areas or hospitals. This should include the nose, throat, axilla, groin and all wounds. If a patient is to be admitted and has previously had positive swabs, then they should be nursed in isolation until a negative result is produced.

All patients with a positive result should be nursed in isolation. They should also commence a decontamination regime which should be available in every Health Trust. Decontamination usually takes 7 days, and then the patient is reswabbed 2 days later. If the swabs are again positive then the decontamination regime is repeated until the results are negative. If the swabs are negative, the screening process is repeated until there are three clear screens. Even then it is not advisable to nurse the patient in the same area as those patients who are deemed to be at risk.

'Soft' tissue injuries of the head and neck

In addition to the obvious skin and mucosa, assessment of soft tissue injuries, depending on the site of the injury, must also include the relevant associated specialized structures. These include the following:

- salivary gland and/or duct (e.g. parotid);
- lacrimal apparatus and eyelids;
- nerve injury (facial, accessory, supra-orbital, supratrochlear, infra-orbital, mental) (see section on microsurgical nerve repair below);
- major vascular injury (especially in neck lacerations);
- loss of function of eyelids or lips.

In penetrating injuries and lacerations, foreign bodies and contamination must be considered. If grit is not removed, early tattooing can result which is extremely difficult to remove later. Underlying fractures must also be considered and treated before any wounds are closed definitively. The patient's tetanus status should be assessed and managed appropriately.

Immediate primary closure with complete haemostasis and accurate restoration of anatomy should be the aim whenever possible. In most cases, head and neck wounds can be closed primarily with acceptable results. The blood supply to the tissues is a major factor in this, and it is essential that the surgery itself does not damage the wound, especially at the edges. Provided that the tissues are alive, even wounds that are heavily colonized with bacteria can be closed primarily using appropriate antiseptic and antibiotics. This is seen particularly with intra-oral wounds, which are all heavily contaminated with oral bacteria.

Principles of initial wound care

DECONTAMINATION AND DEBRIDEMENT

All wounds should be thoroughly cleaned, and foreign bodies such as dirt and glass should be removed. However, over-vigorous debridement or scrubbing can cause further damage. All dead tissue should be excised, and if the wound edges are ragged, trimming to form a straight line may be useful. Persistent infection in a wound continues to stimulate inflammation, delays healing, and may result in excess scarring.

WOUND CLOSURE

Suturing is the commonest method of wound closure. Metal clips, adhesive tapes and glues are also available, and are more difficult to use but can be quickly applied. However, accurate skin apposition is difficult to achieve, and consequently they tend to be reserved for lacerations involving the scalp. The epidermis and underlying tissues are accurately realigned to eliminate 'dead' space beneath the surface. A well-opposed *everted* wound edge is the aim, to compensate for distortion following wound contracture.

Suturing and suture removal

When carried out correctly this gives excellent cosmetic results. Many different sutures are now available, but they are generally classified as one of two categories:

- absorbable – catgut, polyglactin (Vicryl) and polyglycolic acid (Dexon);
- non-absorbable – silk, nylon and prolene.

They may also be classified according to structure, as monofilament, twisted or braided. Monofilament sutures minimize infection, produce less tissue reaction and are the suture of choice for skin. Braided sutures (e.g. silk) have plaited strands which provide secure knots but may entrap material, providing a focus for infection. Traditionally silk has been used for routine suturing in the mouth, as it is easy to handle, strong, and the ends are comfortable for the patient. However, Vicryl is also popular, particularly since it resorbs and does not need to be removed. Catgut is also a popular choice, but is not as easy to tie, and tends to absorb moisture and unravel. The final choice oftens depends on the preference of the surgeon.

Sutures placed in the face and neck tend to be removed at around 5 days, or earlier in delicate tissues. 'Cross-hatching' of a scar occurs as a result of closing the wound under tension. Ischaemia of the deeper tissues damages the skin and stimulates excess collagen formation. Such scars are difficult to improve, and are best dealt with by excision and primary closure. Early removal and *continued support* with steristrips reduces the likelihood of scarring as a result of the sutures themselves. Subcuticular sutures may be kept in place for longer, as scarring is less likely. In the case of large neck incisions (e.g. thyroidectomy, neck dissection), sutures are often retained for longer (7–10 days). Scalp sutures are similarly left for 7–10 days, or absorbable ones are used instead. In patients with poor wound healing (e.g. those on steroids, with malignancy, infection or cachexia), the sutures may need a longer period. Absorbable sutures are useful for deep stitches, either as part of a layered closure or for subcuticular skin closure.

Major tissue loss

This is relatively uncommon but may be seen, for example, following attempted suicide, road traffic accidents or industrial accidents. With such injuries there are often significant underlying bony, brain or ocular injuries, and these may also need to be dealt with prior to soft tissue reconstruction. However, occasionally only the soft tissues are involved, e.g. following scalp avulsions. With the use of microsurgical techniques many defects can now be either reconstructed using 'free flaps' (see Chapter 12) or in selected cases (e.g. scalp avulsions) the tissues can be replaced and the circulation restored by vessel anastamosis.

Repair or reconstruction depend on many variables. Associated injuries may take priority and shock may need treatment. Early repair is ideal, especially with avulsed tissue. However, if there is gross swelling or contamination, a delayed approach may be necessary. Following initial debridement the wound needs to be protected and dressed until it is reconstructed. Local flaps are often useful where tissue loss is not great, and has the advantage that the tissue used is similar in colour, texture, etc., to the lost tissues (e.g. Abbe flap for lip reconstruction). For elective reconstructions, tissue expansion can be useful (see below). However, where the defect is large, larger flaps may be necessary. These can be either pedicled or free flaps, depending on the defect and general condition of the patient. Where necessary, bone can also be raised with the flap in cases where bony defects are present (e.g. mandible).

Tissue expansion

Tissue expanders are inflatable bags with an injection port, placed under the skin, most commonly the scalp (Fig. 4.1). Repeated injections of saline into the bag progressively distend it, and the surrounding skin stretches and regrows to adapt. This provides a surplus of skin which, after removal of the expander, can then be used in local reconstructions. The advantages of this technique include:

- similar appearance and texture;
- retention of sensations;
- limitation of surgery and scarring to one region.

This technique has proved successful for expanding scalp skin to reduce traumatic alopecia (hair loss), and for ear reconstruction. However, the procedure is not without complications. Expansion of neck skin may produce pressure on the deep structures, and expansion of the scalp causes a reciprocal depression in the underlying skull.

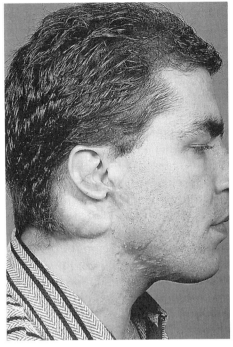

Figure 4.1 Tissue expansion of retro-auricular tissue. This will provide additional skin to enable reconstruction of the ear.

Local skin flaps

Where a small amount of tissue has been lost, local skin flaps may be used to close the defect. Closure under tension may not only break down or result in a stretched scar, but may also distort nearby structures such as the lips, nose, etc. Many flap designs have been described and make use of the fact that there is often a little excess skin on the face which is highly vascular, is elastic to a degree and can therefore be undermined and used to close nearby defects. Well-defined 'axial flaps' (e.g. glabellar flap, nasolabial flap) may be raised, based on a small pedicle through which the feeding vessels pass. So long as these are preserved and not kinked during rotation of the flap, quite large skin areas can be used to facilitate tissue closure. However, random pattern flaps require a broad attachment at the base if necrosis is to be avoided. In contrast to the remainder of the body, the skin of the head and neck is very well vascularized and the success rate of local flaps is generally very high. These techniques are particularly useful in the reconstruction of nasal tips, eyelids and lips.

Parotid injuries

Lacerations along the side of the face must be carefully assessed in order to exclude injuries to the parotid gland, parotid duct and, most importantly, the facial nerve. Injuries to the duct and nerve must be repaired, often using microsurgical techniques, before the skin is closed. Failure to repair the duct may result in the formation of a 'sialocele' which will eventually drain through the wound, resulting in a salivary fistula. Failure to repair the nerve may result in various degrees of facial weakness.

Microsurgical nerve repair

Repair of damaged or severed nerves in selected cases is now possible with the use of the operating microscope. Both direct suturing of the cut ends or 'interpositional' nerve grafting may be carried out depending on the type of injury. Good results have been obtained following reconstruction or repair of the accessory and facial nerves. However, reconstruction of sensory nerves has a lower success rate, but is still often of benefit to the patient. In long-standing cases of facial palsy with atrophy of the facial muscles, free flaps of muscle with their associated nerves and vessels have been used. Ideally early repair (within 24 h) is preferable and should be carrried out if there is no infection or significant associated soft tissue trauma. In the case of the facial nerve, successful late repair is limited by wasting of the facial muscles, which occurs around 6–12 months after injury.

Examples of nerve injuries which may benefit from exploration and repair include the following.

- *Facial nerve*. This nerve may be damaged following trauma or surgery to the parotid region. If necessary, immediate repair can be delayed and at the time of wound closure the nerve endings marked with sutures. Reconstruction may also be undertaken in cases involving malignant tumours of the parotid gland, which require sacrifice of the facial nerve.
- *Accessory nerve*. Injury to this nerve may occur following trauma, lymph-node biopsies or radical neck dissection. Loss of function of the trapezius muscle results in limitations of shoulder motion.
- *Lingual nerve*. This nerve supplies sensation and taste to the anterior two-thirds of the tongue. It may be damaged during surgical removal of a lower third molar. Ideally repair is undertaken within 6 months after injury.
- *Inferior alveolar nerve*. Injury may occur following wisdom tooth removal, orthognathic surgery, tumour resection, fracture fixation or placement of implants. This can result in numbness of 'dysaesthesia' in the lower teeth, the lower lip and the chin. This should be reconstructed within 3 to 4 weeks after injury.

Since the facial and accessory nerves are purely motor nerves and the lingual and inferior alveolar nerves are mostly sensory nerves, repair can be simply carried out by alignment of the nerve stumps or by nerve grafting. Manipulation of the nerves must be kept to a minimum, as this stimulates scar tissue at the suture site, which can prevent nerve growth. It is essential that there is no tension across the repair. The smallest number of sutures consistent with accurate alignment is used. Where grafting is required the great auricular and sural nerves are often used.

FACIAL REANIMATION

In longstanding cases of facial palsy where direct repair or nerve grafting is not possible, hypoglossal–facial nerve anastomosis may be carried out. This provides some tone to the facial muscles, and symmetry of the mouth. Voluntary movements are limited. Other techniques include using the opposite uninjured facial nerve (cross-face anastomosis), making a long graft running through the upper lip. On the non-paralysed side this is anastomosed to peripheral branches, which are then connected to the corresponding branches of the compromised side. Success rates vary, but are particularly poor in patients with facial palsy of duration longer than 12 months, when severe wasting of the facial muscles has occurred. In general, no cross-over procedures are as successful as early end-to-end repairs.

Surgical drains

Drains in the head and neck are generally used to provide drainage of infected material (incision and drainage of an abscess), to prevent the collection of blood or fluid between two large raw surfaces (following neck dissection, coronal flap), or where a large potential space for blood to collect exists and cannot be closed (e.g. following removal of submandibular gland). Drains should not be used as a substitute for poor surgical technique, and haemostasis should be established before wounds are closed. However, 'reactive' haemorrhage can occur, i.e. as the patient recovers from the anaesthetic their blood pressure rises and previously closed vessels may open and bleeding may restart. This probably happens to a minor degree in all patients, and draining the small amount of blood that is released prevents the formation of haematomas which may become infected.

Drains may be left protruding from the skin and simply covered with an absorbent dressing (e.g. following abscess drainage). Fluids drain under gravity. Alternatively they may be connected to a vacuum container. If the wound is not airtight, or there is persistent accumulation of fluid, but it is felt inappropriate to re-explore the wound, the drains may be placed on continuous low-pressure suction.

'Shortening a drain' involves withdrawing it little by little to enable the cavity to seal up gradually whilst still allowing fluids to drain. This is rarely necessary following head and neck surgery, as most drains are usually quite small. However, it may be of use after incision and drainage of an extensive abscess (e.g. Ludwig's angina), to prevent further collection of pus.

Skin grafts

A skin graft is a segment of dermis and epidermis that is raised from its supporting tissues and which can then be transferred to another area of the body. Skin may be used:

- following excision of skin lesions, e.g. BCCs, as an alternative to local flaps;
- following resection of intra-oral tissues to provide a new lining (e.g. tongue, maxilla);
- following sulcus-deepening procedures to aid denture retention;
- palatal skin may be harvested to reconstruct the lower eyelid;
- to close the defect following harvesting of radial forearm free flap.

There are two types of skin grafts.

Split skin graft ('partial thickness' or SSG)

This consists of the epidermis and the upper portion of the dermis. Common sites of donor areas for SSGs are the thighs, buttocks and upper arms. The appearance of the donor site following harvesting is not unlike that of a graze or abrasion. The size and depth depend on the area to be grafted. The donor site can take up to 14 days to heal, as the epidermis regenerates from epithelium lining the sweat glands, hair follicles and sebaceous glands in the exposed deeper dermis.

Donor sites are usually dressed with an alginate and then a film dressing to provide a moist, warm environment to aid epithelialization. This is also more comfortable for the patient, as exposed nerve endings are kept moist. Donor sites are usually more painful than the site which is grafted. Once healed, the donor site will be covered in a flaky kerantinized layer of skin. This needs to be creamed or oiled with emollient cream, vitamin E oil or a mixture of essential oils. Moisturizing should be carried out at least twice a day, with the area being washed with a non-perfumed soap prior to application of the cream or oil. Sebaceous function can be affected in the donor site when the skin is harvested, but does recover over a period of several months. Moisturizing should continue for that length of time. In addition, moisturizing and massage may prevent the site from becoming thick and raised with hypertrophic scarring. The colour of the donor site will vary from deep purple to red in the first instance, and once healed the colour is often affected by the air temperature. This deep colour will fade with time, leaving the donor site slightly paler than the normal skin.

Full-thickness graft (FTG)

These are often known as Wolfe grafts. A FTG consists of the epidermis and the full thickness of the dermis. Common donor sites for FTGs are the abdomen, pre-auricular or post-auricular regions, supraclavicular area and the groin. The area used as the donor site depends on the area to be grafted. Pre- or post-auricular areas are particularly useful for the face, as skin texture and colour are a better match. FTG donor sites are usually directly closed as the grafts tend to be for small areas. Donor sites on the abdomen can usually be closed easily. The time when the sutures are removed depends on the area from which the skin is taken. As with split skin grafts it is recommended that the scar is massaged with cream or oils to prevent hypertrophic scarring and to help the scar to mature to be flat and pale.

How does the skin take?

When the graft comes into contact with the wound bed of the recipient site it starts to absorb a plasma-like fluid. A network of fibrin forms between the graft and the wound bed which holds the graft in place. Fluid is absorbed into the graft over the first 48 h. After this time, blood begins to flow into the graft and the plasma-like fluid drains away. This process is known as 'plasmatic inhibition'. Vascular buds grow into the fibrin network (angiogenesis) forming a new vascular network. A lymphatic network is established by 4 or 5 days after placement, so aiding drainage.

Good contact between the graft and the wound bed is essential for survival of the graft. The following factors can cause failure of a graft:

- poor blood supply in the recipient site, i.e. the wound not being properly debrided down to a bleeding bed;
- haematoma or seroma collecting between the recipient bed and the graft;
- movement;
- infection, especially with beta-haemolytic *Streptococcus* A;
- poorly placed grafts (wrinkling or stretched too tightly).

It is therefore essential that the correct conditions for the successful take are achieved. This can be aided by the following measures:

- delaying grafting if there is excessive bleeding at the time of surgery;
- meshing or perforating the graft so that any excess exudate can seep through the perforations so as not to lift the graft off the wound bed;
- toileting the graft regularly to express any haematoma or seroma;
- the use of tie-over dressings, which are foam or wool dressings placed on top of the graft and sutured into place. These gently press the graft into place, so preventing the graft from lifting off. They are used on areas such as the face and other areas where gravity may encourage separation.

Skin can be stored for up to 21 days after harvesting, but must be stored at 4°C. The harvested skin is moistened with saline and placed on a paraffin gauze and then in a glass jar for storage. The jar is labelled with the patient's details and the time and date of harvesting. The longer the skin is stored the less likely it is to vascularize, so it should be applied as soon as possible after harvesting.

How to apply skin

Most grafting is carried out in the operating theatre at the time of harvesting. However, there are occasions when late application is required, e.g. delayed grafting or when a portion of a graft has failed. The site to be grafted must be clean and moist, but not excessively so. It should not readily bleed, but must have a healthy appearance, i.e. with no slough or debris present. The harvested skin has a moist or shiny side, and it is this side which must be placed on to the wound bed. Any air or fluid should be expressed from underneath the graft. It may also be necessary to perforate the skin at intervals with a scalpel if it has not been previously meshed or perforated. It is important to ensure that the skin lies flush with the wound bed, and to overlap some graft on to the skin edges. Some shrinkage will occur, and this will ensure that the graft takes at the periphery of the wound. A firm dressing is applied if the graft is not to be nursed exposed. This immobilization prevents slippage of the graft. Wool and crepe bandage may be used to support the graft. The dressing is left in place for 5 days unless toileting is required. It is then inspected and the amount of graft take is estimated.

Grafts placed within the mouth are often sutured in place but otherwise left undisturbed. 'Tacking' sutures may be placed to assist in their support. If skin is to be placed over a bony surface (e.g. mandible, maxilla), a dressing plate can be made pre-operatively to cover the area and provide support and protection. With care the patient may be able to eat sloppy food soon afterwards, but only if excellent oral hygiene can be maintained. Dressing plates may be required for many weeks in some instances to reduce distortion of the sulci around the jaws by scarring, which may prevent denture-wearing or oral hygiene.

The appearance of a graft will vary according to its thickness and the donor site. It can range from purple to deep or pale pink in colour. The choice of donor site is therefore important if grafting to the face is necessary. As the graft matures over several months its colour will change and should become more like the colour of the surrounding skin. SSGs that have been meshed will always have a meshed appearance, even when mature. For this reason they are not normally used on areas such as the face.

Care of skin grafts

If all goes well, after 2 to 3 weeks the graft should be stable enough to require no further dressings. It is then cared for in the same way as the donor site, i.e. washed twice a day with a non-perfumed soap and massaged with oil or cream.

Scars

All wounds that extend deeper than the epidermis heal with scarring. The aim is to minimize this to cosmetically and functionally acceptable levels. In uninjured skin, collagen synthesis and breakdown are balanced. However, during healing there is a marked increase in collagen production. This reaches a maximum at around 1 month, and then falls slowly to pre-injury levels. Early on the scar is red, hard and sometimes itches. Any temptation to try and improve the scar before maturation must be resisted. However, improvements in its appearance can be achieved by regular wound massage with a moisturizing cream which encourages breakdown of collagen. It takes about 9–12 months for a scar to mature, during which time significant improvements in appearance can be achieved. The wound eventually becomes less vascular, and softens and flattens. Scarring is due to an excess of collagen in the proximity of the wound.

The following factors promote poor scars:

- healing by secondary intention;
- healing of wounds under tension;
- continuing tension on a maturing scar;
- poor vascularity (e.g. diabetes, irradiation);
- dead tissue, (e.g. crushed);
- linear wounds running perpendicular to crease lines or linear lines (Fig. 4.2).

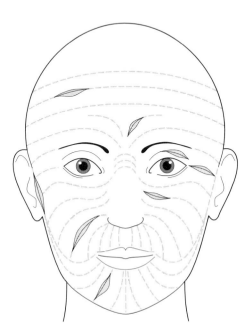

Figure 4.2 Various elliptical excisions of lesions are demonstrated. In general these should be placed parallel to the relaxed skin tension lines (RSTLs) to avoid tension.

Hypertrophic scars and keloids

In some cases scar tissue continues to thicken. A hypertrophic scar remains confined to the wound closure and may soften and flatten after several years (Fig. 4.3). However, a keloid continues to overgrow and may involve previously undamaged tissue. Keloids can become very bulky. The difference between the two types is one of extent rather than structure. Keloids occur more commonly among blacks than whites, and are often seen after burns. In the early stages massage with a moisturizer maintains the suppleness of the scar. Regular intralesional steroid injection (with Triamicinolone acetonide) over 3 to 4 months may be useful for rapidly growing keloids. Alternatively, steroids may be applied topically (Haelan tape). Sustained pressure on the scar has been shown to improve flattening and softening. However, this must be continuous and maintained for 6 months to be of any use. Face masks have been designed and are of most use in burns patients. Surgical excision may be necessary for very large keloids, but there is a high incidence of recurrence. Radiotherapy was employed in the past, but is now no longer used because of the risk of radiation-induced cancer.

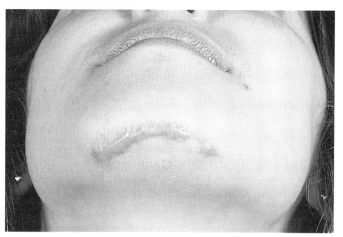

Figure 4.3   Hypertrophic scar formation following a simple laceration.

Management of established scars

This depends on the particular characteristics of the scar:

- *shortened scars* – scars contract during maturation, and may distort adjacent structures, particularly around the mouth, the base of the nose and the eyes. Lengthening of the scar may be carried out by rearrangement using a technique of 'Z-plasty';
- *shelf scars* – semicircular scars contract unequally along each side, and the inner part often bulges over the outer (pin-cushioning). This is difficult to correct, but may be improved by increasing its length using multiple Z-plasties;

- *widened or stretched scars* – tension across the wound or repeated movement can lead to this type of scar, which can be excised and resutured. Supporting the wound with adhesive tape (e.g. steristrips or subcuticular suture) during the first month will minimize recurrence;
- *tattooing* – this occurs following inadequate removal of grit, etc. at the time of primary closure. Dermabrasion or excision and primary closure are the best methods of removing tattooed tissue;
- *badly aligned scars* – scars running in natural skin creases are less noticeable than those running across them. Some scars may therefore be realigned using a Z-plasty, changing the direction of the scar by 90 degrees;
- *uneven scars* – these can be improved by multiple interdigitating flaps ('W'-plasty, 'geometric broken line closure') following excision of the scar. By creating irregularities in the new scar, this breaks up the straight-line appearance.

5 Pain control

Lesley Boys and Michael Perry

Anatomy and physiology of pain

Receptors that are sensitive to noxious stimuli (heat, pressure, pricks, cuts, etc.) release substances such as bradykinin, prostaglandins and H^+ ions. These substances act on receptor sites, stimulating impulses in the nerve. Two types of pain fibres are involved in relaying impulses:

- A-delta ('fast' pain) fibres – these transmit information quickly and are responsible for the acute sense of pain (sharp, pricking);
- C-type ('slow' pain) fibres – these transmit impulses slowly and are associated with dull, aching, nagging pain.

These fibres synapse in the dorsal horn of the spinal cord where impulses are relayed to the midbrain and the thalamus via the spinothalamic and anterolateral tracts. Inhibitory impulses pass via the dorsal horn, whilst other fibres activate enkephalin release, inhibiting relay. Melzack and Wall (1965) proposed that the central transmission of pain impulses is influenced by a 'spinal gate' (located in the substantia gelatinosa of the dorsal horn) that opens in response to an excess of small afferent pain-fibre activity peripherally. Increased activity in large sensory (non-pain) fibres is thought to inhibit pain transmission by closing the gate. Therefore pain impulses originating in the peripheral nervous system can be prevented from reaching the brain.

Since then it has been suggested that, whilst the idea of a 'gating mechanism' may be accurate, more complex mechanisms are involved, such as pre-synaptic inhibition by the dorsal root reflex and certain post-synaptic activity. It is the cortex that discriminates the site of the pain, its distribution and possible cause, and can exert an inhibitory influence with input such as memory, sight and hearing.

Anatomy and physiology of facial pain

The upper cervical nerves carrying pain impulses from the cervical spine converge in the dorsal horn with trigeminal sensory neurones – the 'trigeminocervical complex'. This convergence is the basis of referred pain from the neck to the face and head. Facial sensation is principally from the trigeminal nerve, although there is some contribution from the facial and vagus nerves. The cornea and dental pulp are predominantly innervated by pain fibres, whilst the posterior aspect of the tongue, the tonsils, tympanic cavity and pharynx are innervated by the glossopharyngeal nerve. There is a large representation of the orofacial region in the higher somatosensory system, accounting for the exquisite sensibility of the orofacial tissues.

Types of pain

'Somatic' pain, i.e. that arising from structures of which one is generally aware (skin, oral mucosa, joints, etc.), often subsides following healing. It is usually described as sharp or sore.

'Neuropathic' pain is caused by injury to the nociceptive pathway, and in contrast may persist long after healing has taken place. It is often described as burning, shooting, or like an electric shock. Injury may occur peripherally or centrally anywhere along the pathway to the brain. This can happen following herpes zoster infection ('post-herpetic neuralgia').

One type of neuropathic pain that is often encountered in the craniofacial area is 'deafferentation'. This refers to partial or total loss of a sensory supply to a particular body region, often perceived in a localized area as a result of loss or interruption of sensory fibres. Instead of a loss or decrease in pain sensation in the affected area, spontaneous pain may develop. This is occasionally seen following inferior alveolar or lingual nerve injury (e.g. after wisdom tooth removal). This unpleasant or impaired sensation is referred to as 'dysaesthesia', whereas 'allodynia' refers to pain caused by stimuli that would not normally produce pain, e.g. bedclothes producing a burning sensation. The onset of neuropathic pain may be immediate or delayed, and the nature of the pain may change over time.

Psychology of pain

The complex nature of pain is highlighted by anecdotes of severely wounded soldiers who do not complain of pain, or of athletes who are injured but do not experience pain until the contest is over. The way in which we perceive and react to pain is subjective, highly dependent upon the individual and the current situation, and it may change over time. Nurses need to be able to recognize anxiety and behaviour patterns which may heighten pain aware-ness. Illness and hospitalization inevitably increase anxiety. Previous experi-ence of hospitalization will have either a negative or a positive influence on perception and reaction to pain. Much has been done to improve pain control and the environment for children in the knowledge that the less traumatic the experience, the less likelihood there is of major anxiety problems arising in the future.

Post-operative patients can be classified into three groups:

- those who are panic-stricken and cope badly with surgery, demanding a lot of attention;
- those who show little fear, are calm and confident and who generally do well provided that there are no complications;
- those who are moderately fearful but not overwhelmed, are eager to be given as much information as possible, and tend to develop a framework within which they safeguard their emotions in advance.

Acute pain provokes anxiety, which heightens the pain. Expressions of anx-iety are similar to those of pain, e.g. irritability, impatience, pallor, flushing, and rigid or protective posture. If anxiety is present, the cause should be found and support in developing coping strategies should be provided. If pain is causing anxiety, this should be relieved sufficiently for the patient to be able to cope with the situation in a less anxious way. Pre-operative assess-ment should take these factors into consideration.

For those patients with a diagnosis of a malignancy or progressive disease, anxiety heightens the pain, occasionally to the point of inducing a fear of dying or a wish to die in order to bring about an end to the suffering. Although not all cancer patients experience pain, it is the symptom that is most feared and is the most common uncontrolled symptom remembered by bereaved relatives. The pain experienced by these patients will have physical, psychological, psychosocial and spiritual dimensions. The nurse needs to use effective listening and communication skills in order to reassure the patient that he or she believes the patient has pain, understands their experience of the pain, and that it will be attended to.

Not all patients will 'complain' about their pain. Whilst they do not necessarily experience less pain, introverted or severely depressed patients find it difficult to express themselves and to gain the attention and reassur-ance that they need. These patients need as much attention as those who readily and often describe their pain in great detail. This can be achieved by regular review, good communication skills, support, and the ability to recognize when to refer them to other specialists, e.g. a psychologist and/or a psychiatrist.

Classification of orofacial pain

Idiopathic facial pain represents a significant proportion of out-patient attendances. Four symptom complexes are described:

- facial arthromyalgia (FAM) (temperomandibular joint (TMJ) dysfunction syndrome);
- atypical facial pain (non-joint or muscle pain);
- atypical odontalgia;
- oral dysaesthesia (oral sensory disturbances).

It has been suggested that these symptoms may form part of a whole-body pain syndrome involving the neck, back, abdomen and skin. Adverse life events and impaired coping ability are the strongest known aetiological factors.

The aetiology of idiopathic facial pain is still under investigation. It has been suggested that stress-induced neuropeptide inflammation within the joint causes pain and local production of free radicals. Eicosinoids have also been suggested to be responsible for unexplained pain in non-joint areas, including the teeth.

In 1994, the International Association for the Study of Pain revised its classification of chronic pain. This framework enables us to identify different diseases and syndromes, to compare our experiences, and to facilitate the uniformity of information that is essential to research.

Odontalgia (toothache 1)

Definition: Short-lasting diffuse pain due to dentino-enamel defects. Evoked by local stimuli.

Pain description: Sharp or dull, mild to moderate pain lasting from less than a second to minutes.

Treatment: Protect defective area with a dressing or restoration, administer simple analgesics (for more information see Pharmacology of Analgesic Drugs section).

Pulpitis (toothache 2)

Definition: Pain due to pulpal inflammation, evoked by local stimuli.

Pain description: Sharp, dull ache or throbbing pain, moderate to severe, lasting minutes or hours, with episodes that may continue for several days.

Treatment: Extirpation of the pulp, extraction, combination analgesics, e.g. NSAIDs and codeine, Codydramol.

Periapical periodontitis and abscess (toothache 3)

Definition: Severe throbbing pain arising from the periodontal tissues.

Pain description: Continuous, mild to intense aching, especially after hot or cold stimuli. May last from a few minutes to several hours.

Treatment: Extirpation or extraction, antibiotics, NSAIDs and codeine, Codydramol.

Atypical odontalgia (toothache 4)

Definition: Severe throbbing pain in the tooth without major pathology.

Pain description: Often described as severe continual throbbing in teeth and gingivae, and may vary from mild pain to intense pain, especially with hot or cold stimuli. It may be widespread or well localized, frequently precipitated by a dental procedure, may move from tooth to tooth, and may last from a few minutes to several hours. It may be a symptom of hypochondriacal psychosis or depression, and there is often excessive concern with oral hygiene.

Treatment: Counselling, avoidance of unnecessary pulp extirpations and extractions, antidepressants, phenothiazines.

Glossodynia and sore mouth (also known as 'burning mouth' or 'oral dysaesthesia')

Definition: Burning pain in the tongue or mucous membranes.

Pain description: Burning, tender, nagging pain, usually constant, but may be variable, increasing in intensity from morning to evening. Occasionally associated with iron, vitamin B_{12} or folate deficiency.

Treatment: Treat deficiency states. Often responds to tricyclic antidepressants.

Cracked tooth syndrome

Definition: Brief sharp pain in a tooth, due to cusp flexion and 'microleakage'.

Pain description: Moderate pain on biting, lasting a few seconds.

Treatment: Repair cracked portion of the tooth. Simple analgesics.

Trigeminal herpes zoster

Definition: Acute herpetic infection in cranial nerve V.

Pain description: Burning, tingling pain with occasional lancinating components felt in the skin. Pain may precede or follow herpetic eruptions and last from one to several weeks.

Treatment: Spontaneous permanent remission is common, although the patient may progress to chronic (post-herpetic) neuralgia. In the acute phase, stellate ganglion blocks using local anaesthetic such as Bupivacaine are indicated for severe pain. Transcutaneous nerve stimulation (TENS), capsaicin cream and tricyclic antidepressants are useful.

Post-herpetic neuralgia

Definition: Chronic pain with skin changes in the distribution of cranial nerve V following acute herpes zoster.

Pain description: Burning, tearing, itching dysaesthesias and crawling dysaesthesias in the skin of affected areas of moderate intensity. Exacerbated by mechanical contact. May last for several years; spontaneous subsidence is not uncommon. Prolonged intractable pain of this nature may induce depression and/or suicide.

Treatment: Combination therapy including capsaicin cream, TENS, tricyclic antidepressants and supportive counselling.

Trigeminal neuralgia (tic douloureux) (see below)

Secondary neuralgia from central nervous system lesions

Definition: Pain in the distribution of one or more branches of cranial nerve V, due to recognized lesion (e.g. tumour, multiple sclerosis, aneurysm).

Pain description: May be indistinguishable from trigeminal neuralgia, or be a constant, severe dull pain.

Treatment: Treatment of the underlying cause. A combination of centrally acting drugs such as carbamazepine, phenothiazines and tricyclic antidepressants is useful.

Glossopharyngeal neuralgia (cranial nerve IX)

Definition: Sudden severe brief stabbing recurrent pains in the distribution of the glossopharyngeal nerve.

Pain description: Sharp, stabbing bouts of severe pain felt deep in the throat or ear, often triggered by touch or swallowing and by ingestion of cold fluids. Episodes may interfere with eating and can last from weeks to several months and subside spontaneously. Recurrence is common.

Treatment: Application of local anaesthetic to the trigger point relieves the pain.

Temporomandibular pain and dysfunction syndrome (see Chapter 14)

Rheumatoid arthritis of the temporomandibular joint (see Chapter 14)

Dry socket (see Chapter 8)

Assessment and measurement of pain

Effective pain management depends on accurate assessment. Following a review of pain management services in 1990, the Royal College of Surgeons and Anaesthetists concluded that it is only with accurate assessment that appropriate interventions can be made. Regular pain assessment can be a contributory factor in reducing pain. Since the nurse has most contact with the patient, he or she is best placed to carry this out. Many factors are involved in the experience of pain and the way in which that experience is communicated. Attitudes and behaviour influence the way in which the individual copes with the pain and the situation in which they find themselves. Similarly, our own experiences will influence the way in which we respond to and manage other people's pain.

Simple methods of measuring pain rely on a single dimension, such as pain intensity, which is based on physical, functional or behavioural aspects. Pain intensity should be systematically assessed at regular intervals using a rating scale that the patient understands. The most reliable indicator of pain is the patient's verbal report. Several scales have been developed to measure and document pain intensity and its response to therapy. By far the simplest tools that rely upon the patient's report of pain are Visual Analogue Scales (Fig. 5.1), where the patient marks on the line the intensity

No pain --- Worst pain imaginable

Figure 5.1 Visual analogue scale (VAS).

of their pain, and Verbal Rating Scales (Fig. 5.2), which enable staff to demonstrate the intensity of the pain. Such scoring systems facilitate measurement and recording. These scales have also proved useful for measuring and assessing the effectiveness of management of other symptoms, such as nausea and vomiting.

Pain is assessed at rest and while the patient is moving as it may be aggravated by or present only in response to movement. For instance, the pain in some TMJ disorders may be described as nil or mild at rest, but moderate to severe on chewing or talking. The use of vital signs may be an additional aid to assessment, but cannot always be relied upon. This is because although

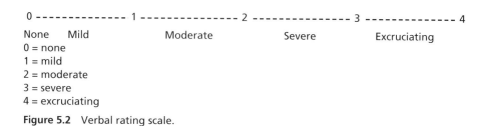

0 -------------- 1 --------------- 2 --------------- 3 ------------- 4
None   Mild   Moderate   Severe   Excruciating
0 = none
1 = mild
2 = moderate
3 = severe
4 = excruciating

Figure 5.2 Verbal rating scale.

patients in acute pain show physiological signs (increased pulse, pallor, sweating and increased blood pressure), some visceral pain may cause the pulse and blood pressure to fall rather than rise. When they are due to pain, these vital signs may return to normal soon after the initial onset of the pain.

Simple tools are usually all that is required for assessment of post-operative pain where the cause is known, and its duration is generally short and predictable. However, when caring for patients with either chronic benign disease or pain due to progressive disease such as a malignancy, a much broader view is necessary. Accurate assessment must include other factors, such as the patient's description of the pain, and any psychological, social and environmental issues which are likely to have an influence.

For more complex assessment, the McGill Pain Questionnaire explores the sensory, affective and evaluative dimensions of pain. It was first described by Melzack in 1975. The questionnaire is lengthy, and is dependent upon the patient's level of understanding of the vocabulary. The validity of scoring and its use in the assessment of chronic pain has been confirmed. However, the adaptation of such scoring systems to meet the needs of the individual is of most benefit. Hapak *et al.* (1994) developed a questionnaire specifically as an aid to the assessment and diagnosis of patients with orofacial pain. It consists of a self-administered questionnaire containing 21 questions, diagrams for showing chief pain location, and a numerical pain scale. Using this tool Hapak *et al.* were able to place 92 patients with orofacial pain into three categories, namely temporomandibular disorders, neurologically based pain (i.e. trigeminal neuralgia, migraine, headache and atypical facial pain) and dentoalveolar pain. It is suggested that this questionnaire may be reliably used to identify patients with orofacial pain that fits any of these categories, without prior knowledge of the clinical diagnosis. Certainly within the pain clinic much emphasis is placed on accurate assessment of the pain description, site, scoring and effect on daily living, alongside detailed medical history and clinical examination, in determining the diagnosis and cause of the pain.

How to carry out a detailed pain assessment

- *Site of pain.* This must be documented with reference to trigger points and/or referred pain. Use a body diagram and date each assessment to determine changes.
- *Description of pain.* This includes the type of pain or sensation felt. Terms include 'constant', 'intermittent', 'dull', 'aching', 'throbbing', 'sharp', 'burning' or 'shooting'. Comparison to previous experience (e.g. like a knife) is helpful.
- *Periodicity.* This includes speed of onset, duration, frequency and seasonality.
- *Influences.* Does anything affect the pain, e.g. movement, heat or cold? Does chewing or yawning make the pain worse? Does the pain fluctuate during the 24-h period? These factors may only be revealed following assessment and documentation over a period of several days.

- *Associated symptoms.* These include swelling, jaw dysfunction, numbness or dysaesthesia, and pain anywhere else.
- *Previous therapies.* Has anything to date influenced the pain, such as analgesics, a change in position, movement, time of day, relaxation techniques or distraction therapy (e.g. watching television)?
- *Past medical history.*
- *Social history.* This should include occupation, family situation, living conditions, smoking, alcohol consumption, employment and hobbies.

For effective pain management, the route of administration is also important in the choice of drug. Patients may not be able to use the oral route post-operatively, particularly after major head and neck surgery, and they will therefore require an alternative (rectal, subcutaneous or intravenous route). Diclofenac suppositories administered peri-operatively will often reduce the requirement for opioid analgesia post-operatively. Combinations of an opioid and a NSAID are used to obtain optimum pain control.

Patients with moderate to severe cancer pain often have multiple pains related to the disease itself, a concurrent disorder or the treatment. Whether the pain is acute, associated with a chronic benign condition or due to a progressive disease, inflammatory, nociceptive, neurogenic and psychological factors contribute to the experience of it. It is therefore logical to consider a combination of analgesics with different modes of action, as well as paying any necessary attention to the patient's psychological needs. Accurate assessment of the patient, combined with a thorough knowledge of locally available drugs and delivery techniques, provides the key to successful pain control therapy.

Assessing pain in children

Several tools are available for assessing pain in children, although difficulties arise in deciding which to apply for each age group. It is much more difficult to demonstrate accurately the degree of pain and the outcome of interventions. An adolescent can report and describe their pain as well as an adult, yet a baby has no such verbal capacity. It is mainly vocal expressions, especially crying, that influences nurses' decisions to administer analgesia. Physiological measures, such as tachycardia, reliably occur in infants who are in acute pain, and have therefore been suggested as a method of assessing pain in infants. However, this response is non-specific and not sustained, making physiological indicators an unreliable method of recording chronic pain. Similarly, the validity of the use of behavioural scales, such as the Children's Hospital of Eastern Ontario Pain Scale (CHEOPS) and the Princess Margaret Hospital Pain Assessment Tool (PMHPAT), in assessing and measuring chronic pain in children have also been questioned. The CHEOPS scale was designed for 1- to 5-year-olds and consists of six groups of behaviour patterns, namely crying, facial expression, verbalizing, movements of the torso and legs, and touching of the wound. The PMHPAT was designed for 7- to 14-year-olds and consists of five elements that are indicative of pain, namely facial expression, nurse's assessment, position in bed, sounds and self-assessment.

In order to assess children's pain effectively, it is necessary to measure more than one dimension of pain experience. The ideal approach appears to be identification of what is required within your own area, and using the criteria that emerge to underpin the development of an individualized tool. The King's Healthcare Pain Assessment Tool for Children (PATCH) evolved in this way. The PATCH tool combines elements from five existing types of paediatric pain assessment scales, namely a faces scale, body outline, numerical analogue scale, descriptive words and a behavioural scale (Fig. 5.3). These elements were found to be acceptable in children with a variety of pain problems. The aim is to assess and measure pain in children quickly and efficiently, so that we can deliver fast, individualized and therefore effective pain relief.

Post-operative pain

Post-operative pain has inflammatory, nociceptive, neurogenic and psychological components. Effective management reduces both the catabolic response to surgery and post-operative complications, and improves rehabilitation, thereby reducing the length of hospital stay. This starts with accurate individualized assessment and continues with careful selection of optimum drug combinations and delivery systems that are specific to the patient's requirements. Support for the patient is also important during each stage of their recovery and, in the event of major surgery, support for the family is needed as well.

The ideal regimen for acute pain should minimize its onset, and provide rapid relief when required, in amounts that are tailored to suit the individual. It should also be simple and safe to use. NSAIDs may be given peri-operatively as pre-emptive analgesia and continued post-operatively to minimize pain due to surgery or trauma and also bone pain. In maxillofacial surgery, whilst the value of NSAIDs in the management of post-operative pain is well documented, NSAIDs alone are often insufficient.

Short-acting opioids such as intravenous fentanyl are commonly used for peri-operative analgesia. A longer-acting opioid such as morphine may be used for extension of analgesia into the post-operative period. In this situation, opioid side-effects may also continue into the post-operative period. It is imperative that the nurse elicits the dose of all analgesic drugs given during surgery, including neural blockade, in order to provide effective, safe, post-operative pain relief. Within the intensive-care environment, the usual mode of administration of opioids is via continuous intravenous infusion. Other more traditional regimens include 4-hourly intramuscular or subcutaneous opioids as required. Provided that the patient communicates their pain and their wish for analgesia to the nurse, and provided that the nurse is able to respond immediately, this regimen of analgesia will usually be sufficient.

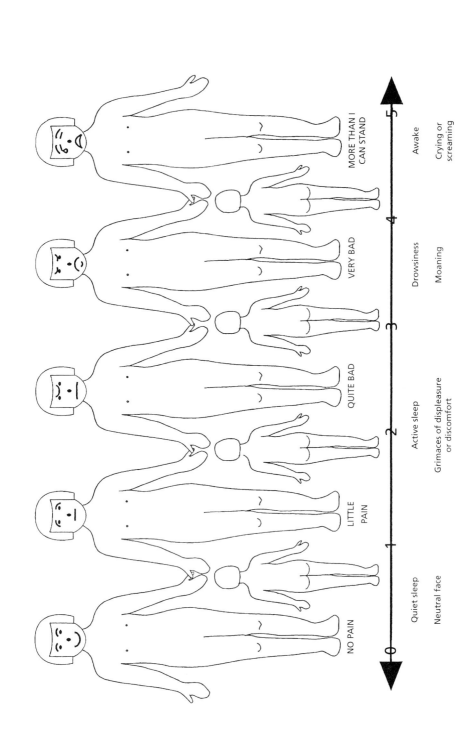

Figure 5.3 The King's Healthcare Pain Assessment Tool for Children.

However, a more successful mode of administration is via a 'patient-controlled analgesia' system.

Patient-controlled analgesia (PCA)

PCA allows the patient to titrate the analgesia according to their pain. In doing this, the patient is more likely to remain within the 'therapeutic window'. There is a strong relationship between the concentration of opioid in plasma and its effects in the central nervous system, i.e. its pain relief properties and side-effects. When opioids are administered as required via intramuscular injection, the patient often suffers periods of intense pain prior to the drug taking effect, interspersed with periods of pain relief, followed by periods of increased side-effects (Fig. 5.4). The use of PCA allows the patient to self-administer small pre-set doses of an opioid, reducing the time delay in administration, and he or she is therefore able to maintain effective pain relief using the minimum amount required, thereby inducing fewer side-effects (Fig. 5.5).

In order for PCA to be efficient and safe, the patient must understand its concept and be physically able to 'press the button'. The programme must be correct and individualized, the staff must be familiar with the equipment, potential problems and how to resolve them, and only the patient may activate the PCA, in order to avoid excessive sedation and/or respiratory depression.

PCA may be administered via the intravenous or subcutaneous route. When using the intravenous route, a dedicated line with an anti-reflux valve must be used to ensure that the patient receives the dose demanded according to the programme set. There are certain advantages to using the subcutaneous route; the incidence of opioid-induced nausea and vomiting is less, and there are fewer line and refill problems. If nausea becomes an associated

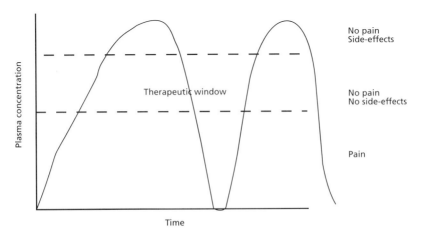

Figure 5.4 Plasma concentrations with nurse-administered 'prn' intramuscular opioids.

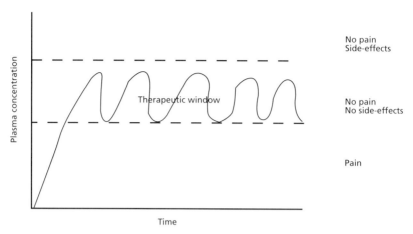

Figure 5.5 Plasma concentrations with patient-controlled analgesia.

problem, an anti-emetic such as droperidol, 5 mg, may be added to the syringe. The usual regimen for patients who are otherwise not taking opioids is morphine or diamorphine, 1 to 2 mg bolus, 5 or 10 min lockout, no background infusion, no 4-hourly dose limit. There have been several studies comparing the efficacy of different opioids in the use of PCA in the postoperative environment, including morphine, diamorphine, hydromorphone, pethidine and fentanyl. In general, although there may be subtle differences in patient response, none of the opioids appears to be superior in the management of this type of acute pain. For patients who are known to be receiving regular opioid therapy (e.g. cancer patients or drug users), the total dose taken in a normal 24-h period must be taken into account when prescribing the bolus dose.

Management of cancer pain

Cancer can cause a wide variety of pain syndromes. However, most cancer pain responds to pharmacological measures, and successful treatment of pain is often based on simple principles promoted by the World Health Organization Analgesic Ladder (Fig. 5.6).

This step-by-step approach can bring relief of pain to about 80 per cent of cancer patients. The first step is to commence a non-opioid analgesic such as aspirin, paracetamol or a NSAID. If the pain persists or increases, a weak opioid such as codeine is commenced, with or without the addition of a NSAID. If this proves to be inadequate, a strong opioid such as morphine is substituted for the weak opioid. Consideration should be given to adjuvant therapy, such as the addition of centrally acting drugs, NSAIDs, and referral to other specialists (e.g. oncologist, pain relief team, or palliative care team).

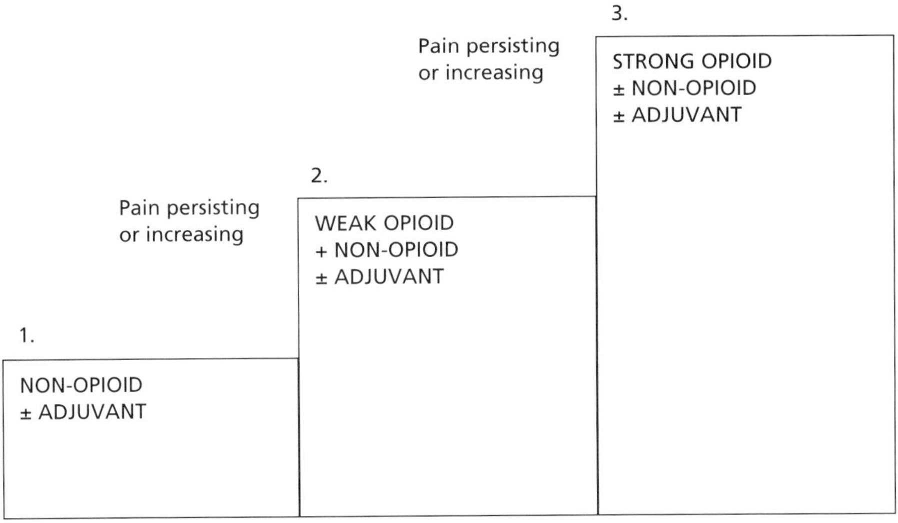

Adjuvant treatment includes radiotherapy, chemotherapy, steroids and psychological management

Figure 5.6 World Health Organization (WHO) Analgesic Ladder.

When commencing morphine the ideal route of administration is by mouth. The simplest method of dose titration is with a regular immediate-release morphine given every 4 h, with the same dose available for break-through pain as often as required. The regular dose may then be adjusted according to the dose of rescue analgesia required in a day. As there is no such thing as a 'standard dose' of morphine, the dose must be titrated against the pain for each patient. If the pain returns before the next dose is due, the regular dose should be increased. Once the pain is controlled the morphine may be converted to a slow-release preparation for convenience and patient compliance. A prophylactic anti-emetic and a laxative should always be given when commencing opioids, as they often induce nausea and constipation.

If the patient is unable to take oral medication, the preferred alternative routes are rectal and subcutaneous. The bioavailability of morphine by rectal and oral routes is the same, as is the duration of analgesia. However, controlled-release tablets should not be crushed or used for rectal administration, as crushing alters their dissolution and absorption characteristics. The subcutaneous route can be used increasingly as an alternative to the oral route, and may be given either by bolus injections every 4 h or by continuous infusion. The relative potency ratio of oral morphine to subcutaneous morphine is about 1:2. Diamorphine is usually the opioid of choice subcutaneously because of its high solubility. For some patients the subcutaneous route may not be practicable (e.g. those with generalized oedema, erythema, coagulation disorders or very poor peripheral circulation). In such cases intravenous administration is preferable and may also be the best option for patients who have an indwelling central line. The relative potency ratio of oral to intravenous morphine is about 1:3. For the management of acute cancer pain and for those undergoing surgery, PCA is useful in allowing the patient to obtain the right amount of strong analgesia as and when they require it, and for initial dose-finding. An alternative to the subcutaneous route is the transdermal route. A transdermal system for drug delivery has been developed for fentanyl, which appears to be both effective and well tolerated. Skin patches release fentanyl over 3 days. However, dose tritation can be difficult, particularly at the start of treatment. When commencing this therapy, morphine should be given as required for breakthrough pain.

Often patients require combination therapy, i.e. regular opioids, centrally acting drugs and NSAIDs. Other useful medical therapies to be considered are steroids to reduce oedema around the tumour, thereby reducing pressure pain, local anaesthetics and appropriate antibiotic/antifungal therapy. Oral candidiasis is common in patients undergoing radiotherapy or surgery for oral cancer. Regular mouth care, adequate nutrition and the application of local anaesthetics in the form of sprays or lozenges are all useful in the management of this unpleasant symptom.

Studies have shown that major head and neck surgery can have a detrimental effect on the quality of a patient's life. The management of pain for these patients extends beyond that of simple analgesic regimens. Anxiety and fear are known to increase both the physical and psychological pain experienced. Patients are highly selective in what they disclose, and show a strong bias towards disclosing physical symptoms, whereas their concerns about the future, their appearance and loss of independence are withheld most of the time. In order to provide optimum care we must consider these factors and be aware of the need to refer the patient to other specialists. The needs of these patients will require interdisciplinary team-working, and the nurse plays a pivotal role in communication and the delivery of care.

Orofacial pain syndromes

Trigeminal neuralgia and atypical facial pain are among the most challenging pain conditions in the orofacial area. It is not always easy to distinguish between these and several other diagnoses, but it is important to do so as the treatment and prognosis differ. All forms of idiopathic facial pain should remain a 'diagnosis of exclusion' – that is, all other causes of facial pain should be considered and, if necessary, investigated for. Occasionally patients with odd pains are found to have significant underlying disease, notably tumours.

Atypical facial pain

Atypical facial pain is characterized by an intense, deep, constant pain. It is often described as a burning or aching pain that is poorly localized in the facial soft tissue or bones. It may be unilateral or bilateral, and it persists for long periods. Other symptoms may include allodynia, dysaesthesia, paraesthesia, tingling and numbness. Some patients present following dental treatment, and their symptoms may overlap those of atypical odontalgia, a possible localized form of atypical facial pain. Psychological symptoms such as anxiety, depression, stress, psychosis, anger and somatization are also common, and it is often impossible to determine which came first, the pain or the psychological distress. An interdisciplinary approach to pain management is required involving different specialities such as dentistry, neurology, pain, psychology and psychiatry. Tricyclic antidepressants such as amitriptyline and dothiepin are most commonly prescribed for the pain and can be useful for treating depression, a symptom that is often associated with atypical facial pain. The specific mechanism whereby these drugs cause an analgesic effect is unclear, although serotonin may be involved. The most common side-effect reported is an improvement in quality of or longer duration of sleeping, which in most patients is beneficial. Other side-effects include dry mouth, thirst, drowsiness, hallucinations, nausea, tachycardia, impotence and urinary retention. Neurodestructive interventions generally lead to a worsening of the pain.

Trigeminal neuralgia

Trigeminal neuralgia (tic douloureux) is described as 'a painful unilateral affliction of the face, characterized by brief electric shock-like (lancinating) pains limited to the distribution of one or more divisions of the trigeminal nerve'. The second and third divisions of the trigeminal nerve are usually affected. Episodes may occur occasionally or frequently over several weeks to months, often followed by pain-free intervals. Patients describe the pain as being like a sudden electric shock, frequently triggered by trivial stimuli of the face, such as washing, shaving, chewing or talking, but the pain may also occur spontaneously.

Trigeminal neuralgia usually responds well to carbamazepine and/or amitriptyline, and a muscle relaxant such as baclofen. Carbamazepine is usually the drug of choice, with approximately 70 per cent of patients reporting significant relief. However, side-effects include drowsiness, confusion, vertigo, nausea, vomiting, aplastic anaemia and liver failure. Patients should be carefully titrated to the lowest dose required to control the pain, and need regular monitoring of liver function and plasma carbamazepine concentration. It is also advisable to withdraw therapy slowly in order to prevent acute psychosis associated with abrupt withdrawal. If medical therapy fails to bring about relief of pain, invasive techniques such as cryotherapy, peripheral nerve blocks, percutaneous destruction of the trigeminal ganglion, and open surgical procedures (e.g. microvascular decompression of the trigeminal root) should be considered.

Other techniques of pain control

These include the following:

- topical capsaicin;
- transcutaneous nerve stimulation (TENS);
- cryotherapy (see Chapter 8);
- acupuncture;
- sympathetic neural blockade;
- cognitive behavioural therapy;
- local heat (*not* extra-orally in infection);
- local or regional anaesthesia (see Chapter 8);
- splinting of fractures;
- radiotherapy;
- hypnosis;
- nitrous oxide.

Capsaicin

This is the active principle of hot chilli pepper and is a substance-P depleter. This reduces the transmission of painful stimuli to higher centres. It is applied topically in very small amounts four times a day to the painful area, and is not associated with any adverse side-effects. However, initial burning or stinging is often reported by patients.

Transcutaneous nerve stimulation (TENS)

This is thought to work via the gate control theory. Rubbing or massaging a painful area, or the application of pads through which an electrical current is passed, stimulates A-beta fibres. This closes the 'gate' by releasing inhibitory neurotransmitters, and pain impulses are diminished at the level of the spinal cord. The result is that the patient feels less or no pain. TENS and some types of acupuncture are also thought to promote endogenous opiate release, thereby reducing the pain sensation. Although the exact benefits of this treatment remain unclear, it has few side-effects and is best used in conjunction with medical therapy such as that described above. In the head and neck it can be effective in post-herpetic neuralgia and other forms of deep-seated facial pain.

Electrodes are placed over the region of the pain or the associated dermatome. By adjusting the intensity, frequency and pulse width, the large fibres are selectively stimulated until the patient feels a tingling sensation. Stimulation by short bursts can cause muscle contractions as well as sensory effects. This has been termed 'acupuncture-like' TENS. The patient response is variable and unpredictable. Although some patients need continuous stimulation, others only need it intermittently, e.g. at bedtime to help them to sleep. Success is partially related to the time spent explaining, experimenting and teaching in a supportive manner and environment. This usually requires the expertise of a pain relief clinic, or a physiotherapist experienced in the use of the procedure. Relatively few good clinical trials have shown significant benefits of this method of pain relief. The results are particularly unimpressive in cases where there are psychogenic and social contributing factors.

The application of TENS is contraindicated in patients with pacemakers, and should be avoided over the carotid sinus. Its safety in early pregnancy has not been established.

For the management of chronic pain TENS can be a useful tool for establishing effective communication with the patient and a trusting and supportive nurse–patient relationship, and for encouraging the patient to develop a more independent life-style.

6 Drugs and dressings commonly used in head and neck surgery

Michael Perry and Caroline Evans

Analgesics
Antibiotics
Antiseptics
Antiseptic dressings
Anti-emetics
Bleeding control
Carnoy's solution
Dressings
Local anaesthetics (LA)
Mouthwashes
Saliva substitutes and fluoride
Sedation (intravenous)
Steroids

It is not the purpose of this chapter to enter into the details of all the drugs that are commonly used in head and neck surgery, but rather to discuss the rationale for their use and to highlight relevant points of interest. The reader is referred to any drug-prescribing formulary for detailed information on each drug.

Analgesics

Other measures used in pain control (e.g. TENS, cryotherapy and nerve blocks) have been discussed in Chapter 5 on pain control. Effective pain relief depends not only on choosing the appropriate drug, but on anticipating its need and ensuring regular administration, rather than waiting for the patient to develop symptoms.

Mild to moderate pain

Simple analgesics such as paracetamol and aspirin are useful in the treatment of mild pain, and in combination with codeine for moderate visceral pain. They can be given either on their own, or in combination with each other, e.g. Co-Dydramol. Care must be taken to avoid exceeding the recommended doses when using compound analgesics and combination therapy simultaneously, e.g. paracetamol and Co-Dydramol.

Non-steroidal anti-inflammatory drugs (NSAIDs)

These are useful in the treatment of pain associated with trauma and infection, and bone pain. They have an analgesic and anti-inflammatory action and act via inhibition of prostaglandin biosynthesis. NSAIDs can be used in conjunction with other analgesics such as codeine, morphine and/or centrally acting drugs. Peri-operative administration enhances post-operative pain relief and, when used in conjunction with morphine, is thought to be opioid-sparing (i.e. pain relief is achieved using a lower dose of morphine). Examples include Ibuprofen and Diclofenac.

Moderate to severe pain

This degree of pain is usually best treated with multimodal therapy and attention to the exact cause of the pain where it is known. Opioids act as an agonist at mu-receptors. Their main action is on the central nervous system. When using opioids for acute pain, consideration must be given to the route and delivery system of choice, e.g. subcutaneous vs. intravenous route; continuous infusion vs. patient-controlled analgesia. For the management of pain due to a malignancy, opioids should be given via the oral route whenever possible, regularly and with the availability of additional doses for breakthrough pain. Examples include the following:

- tramadol (opioid analgesic with noradrenaline/serotonin reuptake blocking action);
- morphine – many different preparations are available, including tablets (Sevredol), slow release (morphine sulphate) and solution (Oramorph);
- dextromoramide – useful analgesia for short procedures, e.g. wound dressing;
- fentanyl patches – useful for chronic cancer pain in patients who are unable to swallow or who are intolerant of oral opioids.

Neuropathic pain

It is important to realize that neuropathic pain such as the pain experienced in trigeminal neuralgia does not generally respond well to opioid therapy, and therefore other modes of analgesia are required. These include topical analgesics and centrally acting drugs. Examples include:

- carbamazepine;
- amitriptyline;
- dothiepin;
- baclofen;
- capsaicin (substance-P depleter).

Antibiotics

Not all infections require antibiotics. Indications for antibiotics may include

- evidence of systemic involvement (e.g. pyrexia, tachycardia, raised WCC, etc.);
- rapidly spreading infection (e.g. cellulitis);
- infections that put the airway at risk (e.g. Ludwig's angina, epiglottitis);
- deep-seated infections (e.g. frontal, ethmoidal sinusitis);
- deep-seated penetrating injuries (e.g. gunshot);
- 'at-risk' patients (e.g. immunocompromised cases, risk of developing bacterial endocarditis, cavernous sinus thrombosis, cerebral abscess);
- bone infection;
- infected fractures, foreign bodies (e.g. miniplates) and bone graft;
- some abscesses;
- failure of other measures to treat infection effectively.

However, these are only guidelines. Each case must be treated individually, the decision to use antibiotics being a balance of risks vs. benefits. Alternative measures include:

- drainage (surgical, posture, inhalations);
- removal of the underlying local cause (tooth, foreign body, graft);
- debridement (dirty wounds);
- local measures (mouthwashes, removal of sutures);
- treatment of systemic factors (diabetes).

In all cases, if at all possible pus or infected tissues should be obtained for culture before antibiotics are started. Subsequent sensitivities will guide the final choice of antibiotic. Many antibiotics are available, and most units have a protocol for prescribing. If in doubt, discussion with a clinical microbiologist is usually very helpful. Commonly prescribed antibiotics are the penicillins, cephalosporins and metronidazole. Tetracyclins and fuscidic acid are useful for bone infection. Occasionally gentamycin or vancomycin may be necessary, but ideally only after consultation with the microbiologist.

Antiseptics

'An antiseptic can be defined as a non-toxic disinfectant which can be applied to the skin or living tissues and has the ability to destroy vegetative compounds such as bacteria by preventing their growth' (Dealey, 1994). Examples of antiseptics include betadine, povidone iodine, cetrimide, proflavin and chlorhexidine.

The use of antiseptics in wound care is controversial. In certain circumstances experimental evidence has shown that some antiseptics adversely affect wound healing, e.g. EUSOL. There is growing anecdotal evidence that iodine plays a role in non-healing wounds, although it is not known why this should be.

Betadine is available in a wide range of products, including surgical antiseptics, skin and wound preparations and oral hygiene mouthwashes. The solution used for wound care is an aqueous solution which contains 1 per cent iodine. It is also available in ointment and spray form and, as previously stated, impregnated into a dressing, e.g. Inadine.

Betadine has been shown to be effective against methicillin-resistant *Staphylococcus aureus* (MRSA), and as yet there is no evidence of resistance to it. It is also effective against viruses, other bacteria and their spores, and fungi and their spores. Because of this, iodine has replaced most topical antibiotics. Patients may become sensitive to iodine, and it should only be used in the short term where there is clinical evidence of infection, although it does become inactive in the presence of pus and exudate.

The ointment can be applied directly to the wound with an appropriate secondary dressing, e.g. Mepitel or Jelonet and then gauze and/or an absorbent dressing. It should not be used on large wounds as absorption of iodine may occur, and again it should only be used in the short term. The alcoholic solution should never be used on wounds.

Terra-cortril ointment contains hydrocortisone and oxytetracycline and is used for the treatment of overgranulation tissue. It should only be used sparingly for a short period. Most units only use it for a maximum of 2 weeks at a time.

Antiseptic dressings

Iodine-based medicaments

Whitehead's varnish is a mixture of iodoform, benzoin, storax, tolu balsam and solvent ether, commonly used as an antiseptic dressing in the treatment of dry socket. It is also used for packing marsupialized cysts and as an immediate post-operative dressing after maxillary surgery. This may be left in place for several weeks without becoming infected, although if it is needed for much longer than this then a change of dressing may be required. When mixed with bismuth (bismuth iodoform paraffin paste, BIPP), iodoform paste applied to ribbon gauze can be used for packing nasal and paranasal cavities. Iodine has a mild disinfectant action on organic tissue. However, it is also an irritant and may stimulate granulation tissue formation.

Anti-emetics

Many types of anti-emetic are available in common practice (stemetil, maxalon, etc.) and the choice is frequently a matter of hospital and local practice. Ondansetron is a useful, although expensive, anti-emetic for resistant post-operative vomiting. Granisetron has recently been introduced for intravenous infusion as an alternative and early results suggest that it may resemble Odansetron, although comparative trials are still needed.

Bleeding control

Oozing following intra-oral surgery is common in the early post-operative phase. It often appears to be much worse than it actually is because much of the 'blood' is blood mixed with saliva which the patient may not be able to swallow effectively at first. Usually packs or gauze swabs are placed over the surgical site at the end of the operation to encourage clotting. These can be removed once bleeding has stopped. In the vast majority of cases, bleeding settles with no further action required other than care of the airway, using gentle suction if necessary. If oozing continues, the packs should be changed or replaced and the patient encouraged to bite on them for at least 20 min. If bleeding persists, the mouth should be rinsed out in order to clear any clots and the surgical site assessed. Bleeding can be dealt with by further suturing or packing the wound with surgicel. Other measures include antifibrinolytic agents such as tranexamic acid. Patients rarely need to go back to theatre.

Occasionally, persistent bleeding following simple extraction is the presenting sign of an underlying clotting disorder such as haemophilia. The bleeding is managed initially as described above, and blood is taken for clotting studies. Clotting disorders should be managed after consultation with a haematologist. Known haemophiliacs often require admission for minor surgery and may be given factor replacement, tranexamic acid and DDAVP at the time of surgery, again following discussion with a haematologist.

Carnoy's solution

This is a toxic solution of ferric chloride, acetic acid, chloroform and alcohol that is sometimes used in the treatment of odontogenic keratocysts. Once the cyst has been enucleated, ribbon gauze soaked in Carnoy's solution is applied to the cavity for a set time in order to kill any remaining cells which could otherwise lead to a recurrence. Because it is toxic to tissues, care must be taken not to damage the surrounding mucosa, etc. during application.

Dressings

Traditional (e.g. cotton wool, gauze and gamgee)

Cotton wool should no longer be used to cleanse wounds as it may leave tiny fibres in the wound which can trigger the inflammatory phase later in the wound-healing process. Gauze and gamgee are still widely used as a secondary dressing to help to control exudate. However, they should never be applied as a primary dressing directly on to a moist wound surface.

Low adherent (e.g. Melolin, Release, Skintact, Tricotex, NA Dressing, Mepitel, Silicone NA and Telfa)

These dressings are not non-adherent but low-adherent. They have little or no absorbency, so a secondary dressing is advisable. Alternatively, they should only be used on wounds that have a low exudate. These can be used in conjunction with other agents such as hydrogels and ointments to help to keep such substances in place.

Mepitel consists of a net of polymide impregnated with a silicone gel. It does not adhere to the wound but is tacky to the touch and so is an ideal dressing for securing skin grafts or for use on burns or abrasions. A secondary dressing is required to control the exudate. The pores are large to allow passage of the exudate, and therefore the wound does not become macerated. It can be left in place for up to 10 days with only the secondary dressing requiring to be replaced. This is beneficial, as it reduces both the disturbance of the wound and painful dressing changes.

Alginate dressings (e.g. Sorbsan, Kaltostat, Kaltogel, Fibracof and Comfeel Alginate)

In the 1800s seaweed was found to be effective in treating sailors' wounds, but only in the last 30 to 40 years has the alginate dressing been developed into the dressing it is today.

Alginates are dry, absorbent dressings made from seaweed which contain varying amounts of mannuronic and glucuronic acid. The dressing absorbs exudate from the wound and becomes a particle-free gel. Sorbsan consists solely of calcium alginate and so gels completely. Kaltostat contains 20 per cent sodium alginate and so retains its shape.

The dressings come in flat sheet form and ribbon or rope form for use in cavity wounds. They are absorbent, and so are useful for moderately exudating wounds. There are also higher-absorbency versions of the dressings, such as Sorbsan Plus and Kaltostat Fortex. These dressings should only be used on exudating wounds, and never on dry wounds.

Alginates are also useful as haemostats. Research using Sorbsan as a haemostat in the treatment of burns and split skin graft donor sites showed that blood loss was halved compared to that in wounds treated with gauze (Groves and Lawrence, 1986). Kaltostat achieves haemostasis by the exchange of calcium ions for sodium ions in the blood (Jarvis et al., 1987).

When applying Kaltostat to a wound it is recommended that it is cut to the size and shape of the wound. If applying Sorbsan this is not necessary, as the alginate only gels where it is in contact with the wound. When using the ribbon or rope versions of the dressings for cavity wounds, it is advisable to pack the wound lightly in order not to cause trauma, and also so that as the dressing gels it expands slightly, so filling the wound.

The removal of alginates should be pain-free if done correctly. Sorbsan can be irrigated with saline to wash it off the wound. Kaltostat does not dissolve and should be soaked in saline and gently removed. Very often the dressings can be removed easily if they have gelled sufficiently. It is best if alginates are not changed too regularly, especially if the wound is clean and non-infected, because they help to prevent or overcome wound infection. It is common for alginates to be used in conjunction with a film dressing, as in the case of split skin graft donor dressings. This maintains moisture and warmth at the wound surface and it also allows observation of the wound without disturbing the dressing.

Charcoal dressings (e.g. Actisorb Plus, Kaltocarb and Lyofoam C)

These products contain activated charcoal which is effective in absorbing the chemicals released from fungating and necrotic wounds. This offensive smell is extremely distressing for patients and their carers, especially patients who have a malignant wound.

Actisorb Plus is an activated charcoal cloth with silver enclosed in a nylon porous bag. The silver helps to reduce bacterial growth which can give off more odour. Kaltocarb consists of a layer of alginate fibre bonded on to a piece of activated charcoal cloth. Both of these dressings can be used as primary dressings.

Foams (e.g. Allevyn, Allevyn Adhesive, Lyofoam, Tielle, Spyrosorb, Allevyn Cavity and Cavicare)

Foams are synthetic dressings of hydrophilic polyurethane. They absorb wound exudate and maintain a moist wound-healing environment. They can be used on moderate to heavily exudating wounds which are healthy and granulating. There is some evidence that Allevyn can prevent overgranulation as it reduces the oedema that is common with hydrocolloids and encourages epithelialization. Foams are low-adherent and are often used as a primary dressing. Since many of them are waterproof, patients can bath and do not require a secondary dressing. It is possible for the dressing to be left *in situ* for up to 7 days.

For healthy granulating cavities, the cavity versions of the dressings can be used and left *in situ* for 5 days before a secondary dressing is required. Cavicare is mixed prior to application and poured into the wound to take up the wound shape. It can be left *in situ* for up to 48 h, but will require cleaning in order to remove bacteria, etc.

Hydrocolloids (e.g. Granuflex, Comfeel and Tegasorb)

These consist of a hydrocolloid base made from gelatine, cellulose and pectins with a backing of a polyurethane film or foam. They are completely occlusive and provide a moist wound-healing environment. Fluid from the wound is absorbed into the dressing and forms a gel. It is advisable to inform patients of this gelling effect, as they are often concerned that their wound has become infected and may remove the dressing unnecessarily. These dressings can cause overgranulation tissue to develop.

Hydrocolloids can be used on necrotic, sloughy and granulating wounds, and can be left *in situ* for up to 7 days. They are easy to remove as they do not adhere to the wound surface, and are comfortable because the nerve ends are bathed in moisture from the wound. Patients can bath with the dressing *in situ* as it is waterproof and acts as a barrier to infection. When applied there should always be a 2-cm margin beyond the wound edge to prevent leakage from underneath the dressing.

Enzyme preparations (e.g. Varidase)

This preparation contains two enzymes, namely streptokinase and streptodornase. It is available in the form of a powder and is reconstituted with normal saline or a smaller amount of saline and a gel such as KY Jelly. Streptokinase breaks down fibrin and fibrinogen and streptodornase liquifies and aids the removal of DNA derived from the cell nuclei.

Varidase is used to debride and clean wounds, especially necrotic eschar. It requires a secondary dressing or a semi-permeable membrane to be applied, and it needs to be changed daily.

Hydrogels (e.g. Intrasite Gel, Granugel, Second Skin and Vigilon)

These dressings are composed of a copolymer starch and have a high water content. Vigilon and Second Skin are a sheet hydrogel and contain 98 per cent water. They can be used on a variety of wounds, such as minor burns and abrasions, and can be left *in situ* for 3–4 days. They are applied directly to the wound and require a secondary dressing. These dressings should not be allowed to dry out or they will adhere to the wound, causing pain on removal. Intrasite Gel and Granugel contain 78 per cent water. They can be used in sinus or cavity wounds as they can be applied directly into these areas. Again they will require a secondary dressing and can be changed every 3 days depending on the amount of exudate.

Hydrogels can be used on necrotic tissue in order to debride the wound. However, they should not be used where an anaerobic infection is indicated. They can also be used on sloughy, granulating and epithelializing wounds.

Impregnated dressings (e.g. Jelonet and Inadine)

Paraffin gauze such as Jelonet is a woven-cotton fabric which is impregnated with soft white paraffin. It is commonly used on minor burns and abrasions, but can adhere to granulation tissue, causing pain on removal. It is also used as a primary dressing over split skin grafts in most areas. However, fibres can be shed into a wound, delaying healing by initiating the inflammatory phase during the later stages of wound healing.

Inadine consists of rayon mesh impregnated with 10 per cent povidone iodine. The iodine is released directly on to the wound. It can be used on shallow infected wounds, superficial burns and minor contaminated injuries. It should not be used where there is a known sensitivity to iodine, and no more than four pieces should be used at any one time. It will require a secondary dressing and can be left *in situ* for up to 7 days. It should not be used continuously for a period of 3 to 4 weeks.

Vapour-permeable films (e.g. Tegaderm, Opsite, Flexigrid and Bioclusive)

These are sterile, thin, semi-permeable, hypoallergenic, adhesive-coated-film dressings. They maintain a moist environment by preventing the evaporation of water from the wound. However, they cannot deal with exudate, so should only be used on superficial low-exudating wounds. They can be used as a secondary dressing over alginates, as the alginate can control the exudate and the film helps to maintain the moist, warm healing environment.

These dressings can be useful for the prevention of pressure-sore formation over bony prominences by reducing friction to the area. They should not be used on poor skin as they may damage fragile skin on removal. Over large areas they require a certain amount of skill in application.

Beads (e.g. Debrisan, Iodoflex and Iodosorb)

These products are also known as xerogels, and are composed of hydrophilic beads or powder which absorb exudate and form a gel. They should only be used on exuding wounds and can be used on sloughy, necrotic or infected wounds. The dressings are available in various forms. The beads are made into a paste or incorporated between two pads, and the powder is available in ointment form or as an ointment slab.

A secondary dressing is required and the dressing should be changed once it is saturated. This can be done by gentle irrigation.

Antibacterial agents (e.g. Flamazine cream and Metrotop Gel)

Flamazine is a hydrophilic cream which contains silver sulphadiazine 1 per cent w/w in an oil-in-water emulsion. It is a topical broad-spectrum antibacterial agent and inhibits the growth of nearly all pathogenic bacteria and fungi *in vitro*. It is particularly effective against *Pseudomonas* and *Staphylococcus aureus*. It is widely used in the treatment of burns to prevent Gram-negative sepsis.

Silver ions are gradually released from the cream, thus prolonging its antibacterial effect. It can be used to treat an infected wound or where it is essential to prevent infection, e.g. in the case of burns patients. An absorbent dressing is required. The cream should only be applied to the wound, and steps should be taken to protect the surrounding skin or maceration will occur. Sensitivity is rare and the cream should not be used excessively.

Metrotop Gel is clear and colourless and contains Metronidazole BP 0.8 per cent w/v. It is particularly effective in the control of odour from fungating and malodorous tumours as it is active against anaerobic bacteria. It can be changed once or twice a day depending on the odour of the wound. As in the case of systemic antibiotics, the bacteria can develop resistance, so its use should be limited to fungating or malodorous tumours.

Metrotop is applied directly on to the wound and will require a secondary dressing and absorbent dressing depending on the wound and the amount of exudate.

Local anaesthetics (LA)

Local anaesthetics work by temporarily blocking nerve conduction, with different drugs varying widely in strength, toxicity and duration of anaesthesia. Once the solution has been injected into the tissues around the nerve, it is slowly absorbed into the circulation, terminating its action. However, the rate of absorption is also related to toxicity, and therefore it is essential to ensure that the needle has not been inadvertently introduced into a blood vessel prior to injection. The 'self-aspirating' syringes that are commonly used in dental practice usually enable this but are not foolproof. The maximum concentration in the blood is reached around 10–25 min after infiltration, and therefore observation is required for the first 30 min. Toxicity may involve the central nervous system (confusion, respiratory depression and convulsions) or the cardiovascular system (dysrhythmias, hypotension and cardiac arrest).

Some LA solutions contain a small amount of adrenaline (epinephrine). This stimulates vasoconstriction, thereby delaying absorption and increasing the duration of anaesthesia. Vasoconstriction also helps to reduce bleeding during surgery, improving visibility. Solutions that are commonly used include:

- Lignocaine 2 per cent with adrenaline 1 in 80 000 (lasts up to 3 h);
- Prilocaine 3 per cent with Octopressin 0.03 units/ml;
- Bupivacaine (Marcaine) 0.5 per cent (lasts up to 8 h with adrenaline), and is especially useful for post-operative anaesthesia.

Each drug has a maximum safe dose (mg/kg), which depends on the weight of the patient and the drug being used. Anyone giving local anaesthetic drugs must be familiar with these dose limits or refer to the British National Formulary (BNF) or drug information leaflet.

Mouthwashes

Good oral hygiene is essential for intra-oral wound healing and should be started as soon as possible following surgery, i.e. the next day. Not only must obvious debris be cleared from the mouth but also microscopic deposits which rapidly become colonized and contaminated. In the early post-operative phases effective hygiene is limited by swelling and discomfort and it is then that mouthwashes are particularly helpful. However, mouthwashes are not a substitute for good toothbrushing.

- Chlorhexidine has good bactericidal effects. It is particularly useful in patients 'at risk' of bacterial endocarditis, and studies have shown that the number of bacteria in the blood can be reduced by mouthwashing *before* surgery.
- Hot salt-water mouthwashes are often advised following meals. They help to keep the mouth clean, provide some relief from discomfort and are cheap.
- Difflam (Benzydamine) may be used to relieve the pain associated with oral ulcers or radiation mucositis.

Saliva substitutes and fluoride

'Dry mouth' is a common problem which can occur with no apparent cause or in association with salivary gland disease, e.g. Sjögren's syndrome. It can be particularly severe following radiotherapy to the salivary glands and oral mucosa as part of the treatment of some head and neck cancers. Contrary to popular belief, repeated rinsing of the mouth with water does not help. It merely serves to wash away any natural mucoproteins which have collected and which are important in lubrication. Saliva substitutes are available as sprays or aerosols which simulate these mucoproteins and aid chewing, swallowing and relief of discomfort. Examples include glandosane and saliva orthana.

Dentate patients with a true dry mouth are at increased risk of developing caries. Dry mucosa is also susceptible to candidal infection. Fluoride supplements are often prescribed and thrush is treated with an appropriate antifungal agent. Such patients need regular dental check-ups.

Sedation (intravenous)

Benzodiazepines are the drugs that are most widely used for sedation. They are metabolized by the liver, and therefore alcoholics and patients on some other medications may be resistant to their effects. Contraindications to sedation include acute or severe chronic chest disease and liver or kidney failure. Elderly patients tend to be very sensitive to sedation, which must be used with caution, particularly in the age group over 60 years. Drugs which the patient may be taking for other conditions may cause interactions. Examples include alcohol, opiates, antibacterials, warfarin, antihistamines, calcium-channel blockers and other sedatives. These do not necessarily contraindicate the use of sedation, but must be used cautiously and the patient closely observed. If in doubt, refer to the British National Formulary for the relevant information.

The two most commonly used drugs in intravenous sedation are:

- midazolam – a water-soluble benzodiazepine that wears off quickly and is often used for out-patient sedation;
- diazepam in lipid emulsion – this takes longer to wear off completely ('hangover' effect), thereby prolonging recovery.

Steroids

Intravenous steroids are often used to reduce swelling following surgery. Protocols vary from one unit to another, but commonly include a dose on induction followed by repeated doses post-operatively for 24–48 h. High doses for a short period do not induce adrenal suppression, so these can be safely stopped without the need to use a 'reducing' regime. Care is needed in the presence of infection, as any immunosuppression by the drug may lead to a flare-up of the infection.

7 Speech and language therapy

Brooke M. Quinteros

> The role of the speech and language therapist
>
> Swallowing disorders (dysphagia) and aspiration
>
> Assessment of dysphagia
>
> Management of dysphagia
>
> Speech disorders

Speech and language therapy is both a science and an art, producing a specialist yet diverse range of therapy. This is especially true in head and neck surgery, where difficulties in speaking and swallowing can have a devastating effect on the patient. Frustration, despair and isolation are common problems following major surgery for head and neck cancer (see Chapter 12 on head and neck malignancy). Patients undergoing surgery have the added misery of suffering the likelihood of some degree of facial disfigurement and altered body image.

Each patient must be thoroughly assessed and a therapy plan designed. A variety of therapeutic methods are available which can be used following head and neck surgery. These range from special techniques and manipulative exercises for the lips and tongue following ablative surgery for oral cancer to counselling patients and their carers to cope with the burden of their communication problem. Nursing staff in particular have the opportunity to help to improve a patient's communication skills and boost their self-confidence. Close liaison between the therapist and nursing staff to promote a patient's communication optimally can only enhance quality of care.

The role of the speech and language therapist

Most patients who undergo head and neck surgery will experience, to a varying degree, some difficulty in speaking and swallowing. It is the role of the speech and language therapist to provide every patient with the best possible form of communication system and the safest method of swallowing. He or she is part of a multidisciplinary team and needs to liaise closely with all of the other members. Early referral is paramount and a patient should be seen *pre-operatively*, as well as immediately post-operatively with regular follow-up after discharge from the hospital.

Speech and swallowing disorders may arise in:

- congenital anomalies such as cleft lip and cleft palate;
- head and neck tumours;
- head and neck trauma.

The pre-operative visit

The pre-operative visit is a delicate, skilled session that aims to help patients to prepare for possible speech and/or swallowing difficulties. It is an invaluable opportunity to try to allay some of their anxieties by reassuring them that an expert will help them to manage these problems. This is an ideal time to get to know the patient and their relatives or carers. Listening carefully and establishing a good rapport will help to forge a positive therapeutic alliance. If appropriate, the therapist may supply the patient with a picture chart, erase-board or pen and pad as alternative means of communication.

Following surgery

Therapy begins as soon as the patient is physically stable. The therapist visits the patient in intensive care, advising on swallowing and communication management and tracheostomy care if speaking valves or tubes are needed. Regular therapy continues both as an in-patient and as an out-patient for as long as the therapist deems appropriate. Wherever possible the therapist includes the relatives, advising and supporting them on how best to cope with the patient's communication and feeding difficulties.

Common functional problems following major head and neck surgery

These include:

- drooling;
- speech problems;
- impaired swallowing;
- loss of taste;
- problems with nutrition.

Drooling may be due to scarring, loss of lower lip sensation following mandibular resection, loss of motor function in the lower lip (a complication of neck dissection) or inability to wear a satisfactory denture.

With regard to speech problems, articulation is particularly affected by reduced tongue and mouth mobility. Following maxillary resection, failure to provide an airtight and watertight closure can lead to nasal escape and nasal reflux of fluids.

Both swallowing and speech are significantly affected in cases where the resection extends to involve the soft palate, pharynx or posterior third of the tongue.

Swallowing disorders (dysphagia) and aspiration

On average people swallow once or twice every minute to clear saliva and mucus from the oropharynx and nasopharynx. Swallowing lasts approximately 1 s. Dysphagia, even when only mild or intermittent, affects the ability to enjoy almost all other aspects of life. Drooling and dribbling can lead to psychological and social distress. Just one episode of choking can lead to a fear of eating which, in turn, can lead to social withdrawal and malnutrition. The prevention of aspiration during swallowing is the therapist's chief concern. Aspiration is the intrusion of food or liquid into the unprotected airway below the level of the vocal folds. This can lead to infections of the respiratory system, pnemonitis and pneumonia.

Signs of aspiration

Acute signs (immediately following oral feeding) include:

- distress;
- coughing, choking and gasping;
- respiratory difficulty – wheezing or gurgling;
- loss of voice or gurgling, 'wet'-sounding voice;
- change of colour (greyness);
- tachycardia and sweating.

Chronic signs include:

- pyrexia (fever);
- respiratory problems/chest infections;
- coughing and choking;
- excess oral secretions;
- loss of weight;
- hunger;
- refusal to eat.

SILENT ASPIRATION

Patients with loss of sensation in the larynx may aspirate without coughing and without awareness of the problem. Nasogastric tubes may also be easily passed into the trachea without obvious signs.

Normal swallowing

In order to understand dysphagia better it is helpful to understand first the mechanism and stages of a normal swallow. A description of the normal swallow with a brief outline of some of the problems patients may experience follows.

PRE-ORAL STAGE

The normal requirements are sight, smell, taste and co-ordination.
   Problems include the following:

- loss of smell and taste following surgery and/or radiotherapy;
- xerostomia following irradiation of salivary glands;
- poor posture;
- lack of co-ordination of head, arm, trunk, neck, tongue, lips and jaw.

ORAL STAGE

Normal requirements

Food or liquid enters the oral cavity. Tight lip closure prevents loss of material, and the tongue and mandible function to move the food bolus laterally on to the teeth for mastication. Saliva containing digestive enzymes helps to soften and moisten the bolus, begins the digestive process and helps to provide taste. Typically breathing is nasal and the velum (soft palate) is lowered. The food or liquid bolus is then squeezed by the tongue against the hard palate and moved posteriorly towards the hypopharynx. The velum then begins to elevate in order to close off the nasopharynx.
   Problems include the following:

- ineffective lip seal results in drooling, and an inability to suck, to take food from a spoon or cup, or to initiate a swallow;
- poor tongue movement (e.g. following glossectomy) results in an inability to position food between the teeth for chewing, to form a bolus or to control liquid and propel food into the pharynx. This leads to pooling/stasis of food in the oral cavity, particularly on the side affected by surgery;
- cleft palate or reduced velopharyngeal seal results in nasal regurgitation;
- loss of bolus into the pharynx or larynx results in aspiration;
- poor chewing can result from poor alignment of teeth, dental extraction, soreness, swelling and inability to wear dentures;
- xerostomia or excessive drooling (ptyalism).

PHARYNGEAL STAGE

Normal requirements

This stage triggers the swallow reflex as the bolus or liquid comes into contact with the pillars of the fauces. The velum elevates, contacts the posterior pharyngeal wall and closes off the nasal cavity. The larynx is pulled upwards and the epiglottis tips down over it to protect the airway. Closure of the laryngeal valve system occurs with the false and true vocal folds closing simultaneously. The bolus or liquid moves over the closed airway and passes through the crico-pharyngeal sphincter at the top of the digestive tract.

Problems include the following:

- delayed or absent swallow reflex due to post-operative swelling or reduction in sensation from cranial nerve injury. Mis-timing of the swallow results and the bolus or liquid falls into the pharynx and then into the unprotected airway, resulting in aspiration;
- restricted laryngeal elevation results in unsatisfactory closure of the larynx and aspiration;
- vocal fold paralysis following cranial nerve injury results in aspiration;
- reduced pharyngeal motility results in food and liquid pooling in pockets on either side of the larynx. Food residue can build up on the pharyngeal walls so that food and liquid spill over into the airway, causing aspiration;
- the presence of a tracheostomy tube can restrict laryngeal elevation. Food particles can pool on top of the inflated cuff, so bacterial colonization can occur. Since inflated tracheostomy tube cuffs do not always prevent aspiration, there is a risk of aspiration pneumonia.

OESOPHAGEAL STAGE

Normal requirements

The bolus and liquid enter the oesophagus and are propelled towards the stomach by peristalsis.

Problems include the following:

- ineffective peristalsis hinders the passage of food to the stomach;
- incomplete or constricted cricopharyngeal and cardiac sphincters hinder the passage of food to the stomach.

Note that the gag reflex does not provide significant information about the swallow reflex.

The cough reflex is a protective reflex that is triggered when food or fluid enters the larynx and touches the vocal folds. It may be absent in neurologically impaired patients, and silent aspiration may occur.

Assessment of dysphagia

This requires a variety of both subjective and objective assessments. The consultant's permission is always sought before dysphagia assessments begin.

Subjective assessment

BEDSIDE EVALUATION

This includes a careful review of the medical history from records and observations from team members. A full oral examination and, if necessary, a test swallow of water and soft food is carried out. The blue dye test may be used, in which a few drops of blue or green dye are mixed with sterile water and soft food. A syringe or spoon may be used. The patient may be suctioned immediately and at 15-min intervals over a 1-h period, and the presence of any dye in the tracheal secretions is recorded.

TRACHEOSTOMIED PATIENTS

Note that inflated tracheostomy tube cuffs do not always prevent aspiration.

Nursing staff must be present with suctioning equipment. Partial cuff deflation must be achieved in order to evaluate the pharyngeal stage of swallowing. This will allow the therapist to occlude the tracheostomy tube briefly to normalize airflow and assist airway competence. The patient can now attempt to cough, clear their throat, expectorate secretions and vocalize.

Although the patient may be able to trigger the swallow reflex, silent aspiration may still occur, which will be undetectable. An aspirated bolus may gradually work its way around the sides of the cuff and be removed by suctioning, but the timing and amount will be uncertain. The blue dye test may be used.

CERVICAL AUSCULTATION

This is a technique used to detect the sounds of a swallow via a stethoscope placed on the larynx. The therapist can detect the presence or absence of a pharyngeal swallow and the possibility of a restricted airway.

Objective assessment

A decision to use objective assessments should be made if aspiration or a pharyngeal stage deficit is suspected and it is thought that the results will influence the management plan.

FIBRE-OPTIC NASENDOSCOPY

By inserting the fibre-optic scope into the nares and over the velum, the surgeon and therapist can view the pharynx and larynx before, during and after the swallow. A blue-dyed bolus or milk is often swallowed. Patient tolerance will naturally vary. The advantages are a comprehensive and objective picture of the pharyngeal stage of swallow which does not expose the patient to radiation.

VIDEOFLUOROSCOPY (MODIFIED BARIUM SWALLOW)

Videofluoroscopic assessment of swallowing is a radiographic evaluation documenting the passage of a bolus through the oral, pharyngeal and oesophageal stages of the swallow, and identifying the therapeutic manoeuvres for safe and adequate oral intake. Unlike an ordinary barium swallow, the patient is in an upright position. A teaspoonful of barium liquid and a small quantity of paste of biscuit consistency are taken. Following each swallow the oral cavity and pharynx are kept in view, rather than following the bolus into the oesophagus. The procedure is viewed on a monitor and videotaped. Patient tolerance varies as this is a somewhat strenuous procedure and there are contraindications of exposure to radiation. The advantages are that it provides an objective and complete picture of every stage of the swallow.

Management of dysphagia

When dysphagia is present following surgery, specific swallowing therapy must be implemented. Each patient is unique and requires an individual therapy plan. The therapist must work closely with the multidisciplinary team and advise on appropriate techniques for the individual patient.

'It is important to remember that a return to functional swallowing may take time and that the patient's nutritional status must not be compromised' (Appleton and Machin, 1995). Liaison with the dietitian is vital as alternative methods of feeding may be necessary in the long or short term. If the patient is able to swallow safely but is progressing slowly, the dietitian may recommend a supplement of nourishing foods and drinks.

Alternative feeding methods

Nasogastric tube

This is usually only used in the short term. It can cause the patient discomfort and care is required in placement and in confirming its position. It is usually not retained for more than 1 month.

Percutaneous endoscopic gastrostomy (PEG)

Patients often find this method more comfortable, and recent research shows that patients' weight and nutritional parameters are maintained or even improved on PEG feeds (see Chapter 1).

Swallowing rehabilitation

A variety of exercises may be given to the patient. The full range of motion exercises will not be attempted until the surgeon agrees that is safe to do this without interfering with the healing process. It is not possible to list all of the

exercises a therapist may use, but some general guidelines and helpful sug-
gestions will be given. In all cases the speech and language therapist's advice
on the correct techniques must first be sought. Nursing support and encouragement can greatly enhance the patient's motivation to practise regularly
and so speed up progress. Often specific written swallowing instructions are
placed above the patient's bed.

POSTURE

It is always helpful for patients to sit in an upright and straight position.
Keeping the head up and discouraging the patient from dropping the head
forward greatly reduce drooling and aid swallowing.

Postural variations (after Logeman, 1983) include the following:

- *tilting* the head to the *unaffected* side. This is useful in patients with unilateral
  tongue dysfunction. The bolus should be placed on the side which has most
  movement and sensation. The head should be *tilted* before the bolus is presented, otherwise it will fall on to the damaged side and cannot be retrieved;
- *turning* the head to the *affected* side. This is useful in patients who have undergone more extensive resections, possibly involving the pharynx and/or larynx. The patient *turns* their head to the affected side before placing the bolus
  in their mouth. This closes the pyriform sinus on that side and helps to reduce
  the amount of pharyngeal pooling which may be occurring;
- the flexed head position. This is useful when the patient is unable to hold
  the bolus effectively and/or there is a delay in triggering the swallow. The
  chin is placed down whilst food is presented, thus preventing leakage into
  the hypopharynx;
- tipping the head backwards. Caution must be exercised when using this
  position. It is useful in patients with total glossectomy as it allows gravity
  to help speed up oral transit. Aspiration is increased, especially if there is a
  problem in the pharyngeal stage. To increase safety this technique can be
  combined with the supra-glottic swallow;
- the supra-glottic swallow. This is useful for most neurological dysphagias
  and for patients who have both oral-stage difficulties and reflexive airway
  protection. It can be practised without a bolus. Make sure that the patient is
  sitting upright.

1 Take a breath and hold it tightly (this encourages vocal fold closure).
2 Take a sip or mouthful of food and keep holding the breath.
3 Swallow hard, still holding the breath.
4 Cough out hard or clear the throat.
5 Pause before the next swallow.
6 Remain seated in an upright posture for 20 min after eating.

PROSTHETICS

Prosthetic devices can greatly aid the rehabilitation of swallowing after oral
surgery. They help by narrowing the space between the hard palate and

remaining tongue, and they are known as 'palatal augmentation prostheses', 'palatal lowering devices' or 'obturators'. They are particularly useful when masticating food. The oral cavity is made smaller, so residual tongue movement is more efficient, and they can aid the raising of the velum to prevent nasal regurgitation of liquids and food.

FOOD PRESENTATION

Close liaison with the dietitian, catering department and nursing staff is essential when recommending suitable textures and consistencies of desirable foods. Usually recommended are puréed, thickened liquids and a soft diet, but the levels of consistency must be correct in order to help the patient to swallow successfully. The presentation of puréed food in particular is often the factor that determines whether or not a patient perseveres with their swallowing. Puréeing the individual vegetables and meat separately and using commercially available food moulds to shape the purée into pleasant appetizing food shapes greatly enhances presentation, making the food far more palatable and attractive to the patient. Both the dietitian and the speech and language therapist will have lists and recipe books of suitable foods.

FEEDING AIDS

There is a variety of commercially available feeding spoons, dysphagia cups and mugs, which aid the manoeuvring and propulsion of food and liquid. The spoons have small bowls and long handles for ease of placement. Because they are made of strong, smooth plastic they are less irritating and abrasive in sore mouths, and do not have the metallic taste often experienced after irradiation. The therapist will advise on the appropriate aid to use.

ORAL HYGIENE

Close liaison is required to help to promote the best oral hygiene regime possible for post-surgical patients. These patients often need careful guidance and much encouragement to remember to keep their mouths clean. Swelling, soreness and xerostomia can make this difficult for them.

Speech disorders

Normal speech is dependent upon the normal functioning of:

- the nervous system;
- hearing;
- the respiratory system, including both the lower system (trachea, bronchi and lungs) and upper nasal cavity;
- the oropharynx, including the lips, cheeks, tongue, dentition and larynx.

Language is the message to be communicated, and speech is one channel for communication. Other channels include gesture, facial expression and writing. It is useful to remember that a communication disability is not one person's problem, but that it affects everyone with whom that person comes into contact. Very often during their stay in hospital no one has closer contact with the speech-impaired patient than the nursing staff. Therefore a knowledge of speech disorders and how best to help will greatly reduce the patients' anxiety and frustration, thus improving their quality of care.

Management of speech disorders

Many patients achieve normal voice and speech, but unfortunately for some patients following major head and neck surgery a return to normal speech may not be possible. However, it is encouraging to hear how intelligible even a total glossectomy patient can sound. The therapist aims to achieve the maximum intelligibility possible for the patient by making the best use of what speech musculature remains and, when necessary, providing alternative methods of communication.

Alternative communication aids

The therapist will advise on which aid is most appropriate for the patient. A few aids will be briefly described below.

Voice aids

FOR TRACHEOSTOMY PATIENTS

While the tracheostomy tube is cuffed the patient will be aphonic. When the consultant gives permission to deflate the cuff, allowing air into the upper airway and through the vocal folds, the therapist can manipulate the tube and help the patient to speak. Working closely with the surgeons and nursing staff, a choice of speaking valve or talking tube will be made from the wide variety available. Certainly the restoration of oral communication helps to improve the tracheostomied patient's quality of life.

FOR LARYNGECTOMY PATIENTS

Special voice prosthesis valves can be fitted during or after the laryngectomy. Some of these can stay in place for several months, while others might need to be changed and cleaned daily. Specialist speech and language therapists are trained to size, fit and change these valves. Often patients are taught how to look after their own valves. These valves have to be occluded by the patient's finger in order to shunt air into the pharyngeal–oesophageal segment to produce voice sounds.

An artificial larynx may be provided if a valve is unsuitable. This is generally a hand-held battery-operated vibrator which is placed under the chin. Operated by a switch to control pitch and volume, it provides a pseudo-voice which the patient learns how to shape carefully into speech.

Other communication aids

A variety of other aids are available, ranging from the simple but practical 'low-tech' devices such as picture boards, pen and pad for writing and eye-pointing charts, to 'high-tech' devices such as the canon communicator, lightwriter, switches and computers.

Prosthetics

Just as prosthetic devices can greatly improve swallowing, so they also help to improve speech following oral surgery. The technician may require the therapist's advice on phonology and compensatory speech movements when designing the best possible prosthetic device for the patient.

General hints to help communication

- Find out from the speech and language therapist how best to help each patient.
- Listen, look and never ignore a patient with speech impairment.
- Give the patient time to communicate, and try not to finish what he or she is saying.
- Encourage non-verbal communication such as mouthing, mime, gesture and facial expression.
- Encourage voicing when the patient is able to do this, and praise attempts.
- Always say if you have not understood. Do not insult the patient by pretending that you have, as this is patronizing and demoralizing for him or her.
- Remind the patient to pause between words and slightly over-exaggerate pronunciation.
- Always include the patient in conversation, and avoid talking 'over' them or about them in their presence.

Minor oral surgery (MOS) and oral hygiene

8

Sharon Maddix, Michael Perry and Jo Kerr

General principles
Surgical principles
Impacted and ectopic teeth
Cysts of the jaws
Removal of retained roots
Oral antral fistulae
Soft tissue surgery
Oral hygiene

This section covers a variety of procedures carried out on both the 'hard' and 'soft' tissues of the mouth, the majority of which can be successfully completed under local anaesthesia with or without sedation. Surgery performed on the 'hard' tissues (the teeth and their supporting bone) and associated soft tissues is termed dento-alveolar surgery. 'Exodontia' refers to the simple extraction of teeth using forceps or elevators. Common 'soft' tissue procedures include biopsy, excision of small mucosal lesions, cryosurgery, frenectomy and minor procedures to aid provision of dentures (see also Chapter 16 on pre-prosthetic surgery).

Dentoalveolar surgery includes:

- removal of impacted teeth/buried roots;
- removal of ectopic teeth;
- removal of bone cysts, including periapical surgery;
- closure of oral antral fistulae (OAF).

Even simple extraction of teeth must be regarded as a surgical procedure, and a medical, drug and allergy history is necessary (e.g. bleeding tendency, risk from bacteraemia, medication including warfarin, steroids, etc.) (see Chapter 1). The sex, age, build and race of the patient may all affect the level of difficulty of an extraction. Classically, teeth in partially edentulous elderly patients are described as 'glass in concrete'. Extractions in AfroCaribbeans are also particularly difficult.

General principles

Attending for surgery

For many patients undergoing minor oral surgery, psychological aspects are often forgotten. However, what may be a routine and minor procedure for the surgeon may be a major event for the patient. Every effort must be made to reduce any anxieties. Time spent at the initial consultation explaining what is involved, supplemented with booklets, will help to reduce the patient's apprehension.

Immediately prior to the surgery, the patient should be received in a courteous and unhurried fashion and seated comfortably in the dental chair. Unnecessary outer clothing should be removed prior to draping, as these garments, together with the heat from the operating light and warm environment, may make the patient feel uncomfortable. The procedure and side to be operated on should be confirmed with the patient, and all notes and radiographs should be available. If sedation is to be given, the availability of a responsible adult to take the patient home afterwards must also be confirmed. Reassurance and encouragement are often necessary. In appropriate circumstances, simply holding the patient's hand can go a long way towards reassuring them.

Most procedures can technically be carried out under local anaesthesia (LA), with or without intravenous sedation or relative analgesia (this is particularly useful in children). However, the decision to use LA depends not only on the surgery but also on the patient's attitude towards this and their social circumstances. If general anaesthesia is required, this is often provided on a day-case basis (see Chapter 3).

Local anaesthesia is given and the patient is positioned so that the surgeon and assistant can work comfortably with a good view. Usually this involves the patient being in a semi-reclined position, although occasionally a more horizontal position may be necessary. If this is the case, protection of the airway is essential and may be achieved by warning the patient, loosely placing a gauze swab (so that the patient can still breathe!) just behind the surgical site or using high-vacuum suction. Blood and other fluids should be continuously sucked away to prevent coughing and aspiration. Care is also necessary in advanced pregnancy, as pressure from the uterus on the inferior vena cava can impede venous return to the heart, resulting in loss of consciousness (postural supine hypotensive syndrome).

Good working conditions are essential as the patient is constantly aware of what is going on around them. Faulty or missing equipment and continual interruptions do very little to inspire confidence in the surgeon or his or her assistant. Essential items include the following:

- *light* – this must be adjustable yet not become contaminated by the surgeon's hands. Sterilized plastic drapes which cover the handles, or sterilizable handles, are useful;
- *suction* – high-vacuum, low-velocity suction with replaceable sterile tips is used to remove blood and other fluids. High-speed burrs used for cutting teeth create an aerosol which, if not aspirated, can contaminate the surgeon and their assistant and increase the risk of cross-infection;
- *instruments* – these tend to be provided in sterilized sets or as individual items. They need to be maintained regularly, particularly handpieces, which can quickly become clogged. All chisels, osteotomes, etc., need to be sharpened regularly;
- *assistance* – good teamwork creates an atmosphere of efficiency which maintains the patient's confidence. Skilled assistance is essential, and the assistant needs to be experienced in order to anticipate the surgeon's next step in the procedure;
- *sutures* – traditionally black silk has been used, as it is easy to handle and tie, strong, and comfortable for the patient. However, in many units vicryl, catgut and chromic catgut are now used. The choice is largely a matter of personal preference and cost;
- *swabs and dressings* – most wounds are sutured, but sometimes a covering or pack is necessary. Sterile ribbon gauze, 1 cm wide, soaked in iodoform paint (Whitehead's varnish) or Bisthmus in Iodoform paraffin paste (BIPP) is often used. This can be left in the wound for many weeks without infection developing. Sedative packing materials (e.g. Co-pak) can be used around adjacent teeth or held in position by a plate. These materials contain Eugenol, which reduces post-operative discomfort.

By its very nature minor oral surgery is never a sterile procedure, yet it is surprising how very uncommon wound infections are, despite the numerous organisms that are present in the mouth. However, this should not lead to complacency, and aseptic technique is just as important as in any other surgical disipline. Sterilized disposal items are often used to reduce the costs of recycling. Sterilization techniques depend in part on which pieces of equipment are being sterilized.

- Autoclaving can tarnish, corrode or rust instruments if they do not have a drying phase.
- Dry-heat sterilization is preferable for cutting instruments such as chisels, since autoclaving may reduce their sharpness.
- Sterilization of handpieces is a particular problem. For some handpieces, dry heat is preferable, but they must be carefully cleaned and lubricated with special heat-resistant oils beforehand. Others with sealed bearings can be autoclaved (check the manufacturer's instructions).
- Chemical disinfection – no chemical solution is available that will sterilize intruments without producing tissue damage if drops fall in the wound.

- Hand disinfection – Hibiscrub (4 per cent chlorhexadine gluconate), Betadine (7.5 per cent povidone iodine), 70 per cent alcohol or hibisol (2.5 per cent chlorhexadine in 70 per cent alcohol) may be used.

Surgical principles

It is not possible to outline every technique in detail, and the reader is referred to any standard textbook of oral surgery for this. Here the main principles of surgery will be outlined. These include the following:

- accurate isolation of the tooth/root/cyst prior to surgery in order to plan the surgical approach;
- effective local anaesthetic (with or without sedation);
- access;
- removal of bone (not excessive);
- removal of pathology;
- irrigation;
- haemostasis;
- wound closure;
- post-operative instructions and analgesia.

Peri-operative medication may be required, but this varies according to local policy and for certain 'at-risk' patients. Commonly prescribed drugs include the following:

- local anaesthetic;
- sedative drugs;
- antibiotics;
- steroids (e.g. dexamethasone) to reduce post-operative swelling;
- non-steroidal anti-inflammatory drugs (NSAIDs) for pain relief and to reduce swelling.

Dento-alveolar surgery involves exposing the tooth-supporting bone through one of several mucoperiosteal flaps. When healed these flaps need to maintain a healthy attachment to the teeth, which is essential for dental health. In general, incision lines should be planned so that at the end of the operative procedure the wound edge is supported by intact bone.

After raising the flap, enough bone is removed to expose the tooth, root, cyst, etc., which can then be elevated or removed. Alternatively the tooth may be divided in order to reduce the amount of bone removed. 'Surgical exposure' involves exposing the widest part of the tooth, which then has a bracket or gold chain cemented on to it to encourage normal eruption using light elastics. 'Surgical repositioning' may occasionally be undertaken for otherwise healthy teeth, and in some cases teeth can be 'transplanted' into previously prepared sockets as a form of tooth replacement (in the same patient).

A working knowledge of local anatomy is necessary, as there are many hidden 'traps' for the unwary. Areas of concern include the following:

- inferior alveolar nerve;
- lingual nerve;
- mental nerve;
- maxillary sinus;
- floor of the nose;
- adjacent teeth;
- submandibular triangle;
- infratemporal fossa.

These are all at risk of injury/displacement of the tooth, etc., into them, depending on the specific procedure.

In addition, the surgeon must be aware of :

- adjacent teeth (e.g. presence of fillings, or bridges which may be damaged);
- age and racial variations – AfroCaribbeans have already been mentioned, and in the elderly patient the mandible can easily fracture;
- root morphology – curved roots can prevent simple extractions;
- ankylosis;
- associated infection;
- possible associated disease (e.g. cysts, tumours);
- the presence of other local problems which may affect surgery (e.g. Paget's disease, osteoradionecrosis, vascular malformations);
- the risk of fracturing the mandible or maxilla.

Complications

These partly depend on the specific procedure, and include the following:

- pain;
- bleeding;
- swelling;
- local infection;
- injury to adjacent teeth or tissues;
- nerve injury;
- mandibular/maxillary fracture;
- oroantral/oronasal fistula formation;
- loss of tooth into adjacent stuctures (e.g. maxillary sinus, lung);
- retained roots;
- recurrence of disease (especially with some types of cyst);
- fracture of tooth – not all retained roots need to be removed, and a small fragment in the absence of any symptoms, infection, and in a patient without risk of bacterial endocarditis can be left in most cases. To attempt to remove a root near an important structure (e.g. ID nerve) may damage that structure;

- extraction of the wrong tooth;
- dislocated jaw.

Post-operative bleeding

Most cases need only simple reassurance and asking the patient to bite firmly on a clean handkerchief over the area for at least 20 min. Clots should not be removed unless further surgery to stop the bleeding is necessary, as removal may cause further bleeding. If surgery is required, most bleeding can be dealt with by simply suturing the wound edges. Haemostatic packs such as Surgicel or Kaltostat may occasionally be necessary. If all else fails, the patient must be admitted for bed rest and investigated for bleeding disorders or liver disease.

Dry socket

This is localized inflammation of a socket following extraction, most commonly the lower wisdom teeth. Typically the patient complains of severe dull throbing pain around 4–5 days after extraction, and often experiences a bad taste in the mouth. The pain is often exquisite, with inflammation, exposed bone and halitosis. Predisposing factors include the following:

- difficult extraction;
- pre-existing infection;
- poor blood supply (e.g. Paget's disease, following radiotherapy);
- smoking – nicotine is a vasoconstrictor;
- systemic disorder (e.g. diabetes, etc.);
- oral contraceptive.

The socket is irrigated with warm saline, and is then dressed with an antiseptic pack (e.g. Alvogyl), which contains iodoform (antiseptic), eugonal (sedative) and seaweed (for bulk). This is resorbed as healing occurs. Antibiotics may also be necessary.

Post-operative care

Immediately after surgery the chair is slowly returned to the upright position and the patient is instructed not to get up in case fainting occurs. After a few minutes they can then get up if they so wish. The patient is given analgesics, antibiotics if necessary and written post-operative instructions, which are verbally reinforced. In particular they should be warned that they may well develop bruising and swelling. Because they have been given a local anaesthetic they must be careful not to injure the numb area until it has regained sensation (i.e. avoid biting, hot drinks, etc.). Hot drinks and mouthwashes should also be avoided for 24 h as these may encourage bleeding or dislodge any clots that are present. Thereafter regular mouthwashes (e.g. corsodyl and hot salt water) are encouraged to help to keep the mouth clean. If possible the patient should try to chew on the other side and *gently* clean the whole mouth afterwards with a soft toothbrush.

Bleeding must be checked before the patient is allowed to go home, with a clear understanding of care of the mouth, administering of tablets and what to do and who to contact in an emergency.

Impacted and ectopic teeth

Although any tooth may become impacted, these are usually third molars, canines, second premolars and supernumerary teeth (Fig. 8.1). These teeth may also be ectopically placed. If left untreated, there is an associated risk of developing a number of problems (see Box 8.1) which can progress without any symptoms. Not all wisdom teeth need to be removed, and the decision to do so depends on a balance between symptoms or pathology and the relative risks of removing them (e.g. injury to the ID nerve).

Third molars (wisdom teeth) normally erupt between 17 and 21 years of age, although later eruption is not uncommon. It is often possible to assess the potential for eruption by the age of 16 years on the basis of clinical examination and the use of radiographs. If one third molar needs removing it is worth considering whether the other three should be removed at the same time. Upper permanent canines normally erupt at around 11–12 years of age. If the tooth cannot be felt by 9–10 years this needs to be investigated. Treatment is frequently both orthodontic and surgical. The options include observation, removal, exposure or repositioning.

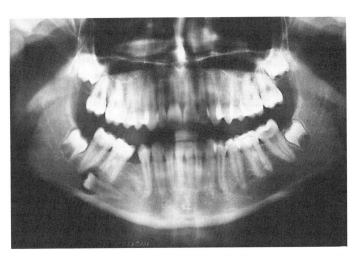

Figure 8.1 Unerupted and impacted lower right mandibular premolar tooth. Note the early cystic change around the crown of the tooth.

BOX 8.1 Common indications for removal of impacted or ectopic teeth

- Pain
- Infection
- Advanced caries
- Periodontal disease
- Periapical pathology
- Disease of follicle, including cyst/tumour
- Fractured tooth
- Resorption of adjacent teeth
- As part of an orthodontic/orthognathic treatment plan
- Prophylactic removal in the 'at-risk' patient (e.g. bacterial endocarditis)
- As an aid to denture provision

An important complication of mandibular third molar removal is injury to the lingual nerve. Incidences in the UK vary up to 15 per cent. Of these, most will make a full recovery within a few weeks, or up to 12 months. However, a smaller group (approximately 0.5 per cent) are left with permanent sensory disturbance. Temporary disturbance of the lingual nerve is often due to retraction of the mucoperiosteal flap during surgery. Permanent injuries often result from nerve division during burring.

The lingual nerve carries sensory fibres to the tongue, taste buds and secretomotor fibres to the submandibular and sublingual glands. Injury can therefore result in loss of sensation on the side of the tongue and the adjacent gums of the mandibular teeth. Most patients describe abnormal sensations, such as pins and needles, tingling or itching, although a few find these sensations painful (dysaesthesia; see Chapter 5).

In selected cases, exploration of the nerve may be undertaken. Scar tissue is released (neurolysis), and if the nerve is found to be injured the segment may be excised and the cut ends sutured together or grafted. The results vary considerably, but improvements have been noted in up to 75 per cent of cases. Timing is crucial. It has been suggested that, in the absence of any sensory recovery by 3 to 4 months following injury, exploration is indicated.

Tooth autotransplantation

This may be carried out to replace unrestorable first molars, missing premolars or upper incisors. 'Surgical repositioning' of ectopic canines is a similar technique. Loss of a tooth results in resorption of the supporting bone. Transplantation prevents this process and is particularly useful in young age groups to preserve the alveolus.

A 'socket' is initially prepared, either by extraction of the diseased tooth or by burring a hole. The 'donor' tooth is then extracted as atraumatically as possible, paying particular attention in order to prevent damage to the peri-odontal ligament (this is essential), after which it is placed in the new socket. The tooth is splinted for a variable amount of time, although small amounts of movement are desirable to prevent ankylosis. Complications include pulp necrosis, progressive root resorption and ankylosis/infra-occlusion. Success rates vary widely from 0 per cent to nearly 100 per cent.

Cysts of the jaws

Cysts of the jaws may be congenital, infective or traumatic in origin. As they grow they expand and weaken the overlying bone, resulting in a hard swelling which may fracture the jaw. If left untreated they can become infected, and very large maxillary cysts can eventually involve nearby struc-tures such as the sinus and orbit, making their complete removal technically difficult. Pressure on adjacent nerves (e.g. inferior alveolar nerve) can lead to numbness. Although 'benign', some cysts, especially the odontogenic kerato-cyst, are locally invasive and frequently recur. For these reasons early identi-fication and removal are desirable. Many types of cyst exist, although those most commonly seen are:

- radicular (associated with roots);
- dentigerous (associated with unerupted crowns);
- odontogenic keratocyst.

Indications for cyst removal

These include the following:

- pain;
- local invasion;
- infection;
- the 'at-risk' patient (e.g. prophylaxis of bacterial endocarditis, immuno-suppression);
- deformity;
- numbness;
- radiographic or other evidence of expansion;
- abnormal isotope bone scan/blood chemistry (can be associated with hyperparathyroidism);
- risk of fracture.

Management

This depends on several factors, including the size, suspected diagnosis, proximity to 'vital' structures (e.g. nerves, orbit) and the general condition and wishes of the patient.

Cysts may be:

- observed;
- radicular cysts (and periapical granuloma) may be removed followed by apicectomy and retrograde root filling;
- removed as described for impacted teeth;
- aspirated or biopsied (where the diagnosis is unclear);
- marsupialized – this involves 'de-roofing' the cyst, removing its contents and allowing it to 'shrink' by bony regeneration. This is especially useful in the case of large cysts in patients who are medically compromised, or where 'vital' adjacent structures are involved;
- resected with surrounding bone (for locally aggressive cysts);
- resected and reconstructed using bone grafts, skin grafts and soft tissue flaps.

Radicular (apical) cysts and granuloma

These are commonly seen with chronically infected teeth where infection has spread from the pulp through the root tip (apex) into the 'periapical' bone. The infected dead pulp in the tooth needs to be removed and the pulp chamber filled with a 'root filling' (anterograde root filling). Following this, the cyst or granuloma is surgically removed by exposing the root apex (after raising a mucoperiosteal flap) and a filling placed in the apex from the opposite direction (retrograde root filling).

Odontogenic keratocysts

These are locally invasive but benign cysts which often recur due to inadequate excision. Once they have spread into the surrounding soft tissues (mucosa, muscle, etc.) complete removal becomes very difficult and often involves extensive resection and reconstruction (see Chapter 12). When they are still contained within bone (commonly found in the region of the mandibular angle) they can be enucleated with marginal resection or curettage. Liquid nitrogen or Carnoy's solution may be used to kill any remaining cells. The patient needs to be kept under regular observation over a long period because of the high risk of recurrence.

Apicectomy

This is the removal of an infected root tip (apex) and the surrounding infected tissues. It is often carried out in an attempt to save the tooth in cases where a root filling is impossible or unsuccessful. It is usually the final alternative to extraction. After anaesthesia has been obtained, a mucoperiosteal flap is raised to expose the bone overlying the tooth apex. Using a large round bur, a small 'window' is then cut to expose the apex and infection. The infection is curetted, leaving a healthy bony cavity. The apex is then cut back and a 'retrograde' filling is placed.

Removal of retained roots

Indications for removal include the following:

- large roots;
- symptomatic case;
- associated pathology;
- causing problems with dentures;
- patient at risk from infection (e.g. immunocompromised or at risk of SBE);
- prior to orthodontic removal of teeth.

Depending on their size and position (buried or erupted), removal may involve simple elevation or a more formal surgical exposure, as with ectopic teeth.

Oral antral fistulae

The maxillary sinus varies considerably in size, and when large can often be seen to dip down between the roots of the upper back teeth. The first and second molar teeth are most commonly closely involved, but occasionally the antrum can extend between the roots of the teeth from the upper canine to the third molar. In such cases, and especially when disease is associated with the root apices of these teeth, the bone is weakened and may fracture off during extraction of the tooth. If this occurs, the sinus communicates with the mouth through the extraction socket (oral antral communication), which may become lined with mucosa to form a fistula. If this is anticipated, the tooth is best removed by a surgical approach so that bone can be carefully removed around the root in order to minimize the likelihood of fracture.

Once a communication has developed the patient is at risk of sinusitis. If the problem is identified at the time of extraction, the hole may be closed either directly or by using adjacent tissue (buccal advancement or palatal transposition flaps). Larger defects may be 'plugged' using the buccal fat pad, which quickly epithelializes. These may be supplemented with a dressing plate fabricated on a model of the teeth. Depending on local practice, many units will prescribe an 'antral regime' to prevent sinusitis, i.e. antibiotics, menthol inhalations and nasal decongestants. Patients should be advised not to blow their nose and to sneeze only with their mouths open in order to avoid high nasal airway pressures.

In the majority of cases most communications will heal. Failure to heal or late presentation require further surgery. Failure to heal may occur in the presence of infection or local disease (e.g. retained root, tumour), and these must be excluded beforehand.

Soft tissue surgery

Biopsy

The usual three biopsy procedures are the incisional biopsy, the excisional biopsy and surface scraping (for exfoliative cytology). All samples must be carefully handled with tissue forceps and immediately placed in a labelled container of 10 per cent formalin solution. There should be at least 20 times the volume of the specimen in the container to ensure proper preservation. Formalin can be obtained from a local pharmacy, together with suitable tight-sealing bottles.

INCISIONAL BIOPSY

This involves the removal of a sample of the lesion for examination. A commonly used method is to cut a wedge of tissue from the lesion continuous with some normal adjacent tissue for comparison. The sample tissue is immediately placed in 10 per cent formalin solution to preserve it, or sometimes it is sent fresh if a lymphoma is suspected. This type of biopsy is generally used when the lesion is large or in a strategic area where complete removal of the lesion would create significant aesthetic or functional impairment (e.g. a large ulcerated lesion on the lip, nose and around the eye). Complete surgical removal of the lesion is not indicated until a final diagnosis is made, since the lesion may not be malignant and may in time heal on its own without further surgery. Surgery before a final diagnosis has been made may create unnecessary tissue distortion by scarring.

EXCISIONAL BIOPSY

This involves removal of the entire lesion together with the surrounding normal tissue. This procedure is carried out on small lesions where complete excision would not cause significant aesthetic or functional impairment (e.g. a small, non-healing sore on the buccal mucosa, where only a small volume of tissue in a non-strategic area is being excised).

EXFOLIATIVE CYTOLOGY

Another method that is helpful in diagnosing oral lesions is the non-surgical technique of wiping or scraping the surface of the lesion in order to collect a sample of cells for microscopic examination. The science of examining shed or exfoliated cells during the scraping process is called exfoliative cytology. This procedure is of limited value and is viewed as an adjunct to the surgical techniques described above. The collected cells must be placed on a glass slide and spread out for examination under the microscope. This slide set-up is called a smear. Probably the best-known exfoliative biopsy is the Papanicolaou smear (Pap smear) that is used to detect disease of the vaginal area. Smears may be taken in the mouth to detect candida infection (thrush).

Common soft tissue lesions that require biopsy or excision include the following:

- ulcers and erosions;
- papilloma;
- fibro-epithelial polyps;
- mucoceles;
- epulides;
- traumatic granuloma;
- benign oral tumours.

Unexplained mucosal lesions which are raised, red, white, pigmented or ulcerated must be biopsied to exclude malignant change.

Pericoronitis

This is inflammation and infection of a gum flap (operculum) overlying a partially erupted tooth, usually the third molar. Treatment involves removal of the opposing third molar, irrigation under the operculum, antibiotics and topical application of silver nitrate or TCA and glycerol.

Cryotherapy (see Chapter 5)

Intractable or recurrent pain from either nerve infiltration (e.g. malignancy) or, more commonly, trigeminal neuralgia may be treated by cryotherapy. The diagnosis must be established beforehand, and this is most easily done by injecting local anaesthetic around the nerve with complete resolution of symptoms. In such cases the nerve (e.g. inferior alveolar, infra-orbital) can then be exposed through the mouth and frozen by the use of a cryoprobe. This can often bring effective pain relief, although this is unpredictable, and its duration may also vary. The procedure can, of course, be repeated at a later date if necessary.

Frenectomy

In children a persistent gap (diastema) between the upper central incisors may be due to one of several causes, one of which is the presence of a large frenum passing from the upper lip to the palate between the teeth. In such cases this can simply be trimmed back under local anaesthetic. Depending on its size, the raw area may either be left uncovered or covered by a temporary dressing.

Pericision

This is simply the incision of the upper part of the periodontal ligament between the tooth and supporting tissues. It may be carried out in order to aid the derotation of abnormally rotated teeth.

Oral hygiene

Over 300 different species of organism have been identified in the human mouth. These include:

- *Streptococcus*;
- *Lactobacillus*;
- *Fusobacterium*;
- *Borrelia vincenti*;
- *Actinobacillus*;
- *Porphyromonas*;
- *Actinomyces*;
- *Candida*;
- *Spirochaetes*;

... to name just a few!

Colonization begins soon after birth and persists for the remainder of life. Even after meticulous professional cleaning of the teeth and gingiva by a hygienist, bacteria are found at these sites within a few hours (up to 1 million/mm^3 have been found after only 1 h). Dental plaque is a firmly adherent layer of mucopolysaccharides, proteins and bacteria which also rapidly forms on teeth and is difficult to remove completely. It is this combination of plaque and bacteria that is responsible for tooth decay, gum disease, tartar and wound infections. Some organisms are responsible for specific diseases (e.g. *Candida* and oral thrush, *Fusobacterium* and acute necrotizing gingivostomatitis, and *Actinomyces* and actinomycosis).

However, despite all of these potential pathogens being constantly present in the mouth, wound infection is remarkably rare and, if it does occur, is usually mild. This is believed to be due in part to the antibacterial action of saliva and the presence of 'growth factors' which aid healing. This does not mean that we can be complacent about sterile technique or after-care, as those infections that become established can be extremely difficult to irradicate, especially if bone is involved.

Oral hygiene is one of the many basic but nevertheless essential nursing tasks, and an important part of daily living. At present it is regarded as more of a ritual than research-based practice. Macleod-Clark and Hockey (1979) stated that 'it is often the simplest procedures that are the most in need of scrutiny, for these are the aspects of nursing practice which are taken for granted and have become formally incorporated into the routinised fabric of nursing. Actions must have reasons and rationales'. In 1981 Daeffler stated that the whole purpose of good oral care was to remove debris and plaque, to maintain comfort and to keep the mouth clean and moist without damaging the mucosa.

The mouth is important for many reasons, including eating, drinking, taste, communicating and breathing. It is also under constant threat of infection from the environment and must therefore be capable of fighting infection. Most people can care for their own mouths, but there are a number of patients who need assistance with oral care. Underlying disease may directly affect the state of the mouth, e.g. painful lesions preventing effective cleaning of fungating and heavily colonized advanced tumours. In a healthy person the removal of food debris is a normal oral function, but this is diminished in patients with ulcers and infections of the mouth. Moreover, in a healthy person saliva is produced in large amounts daily and acts as a mouthwash, maintaining a clean environment. It is also antibacterial and controls the normal pH of the mouth. An understanding of the anatomy and physiology of the mouth and how dysfunction can affect oral health and wound healing is therefore essential. Maurer (1977) suggested that 'an oral assessment should be made on admission, which will then enable us to evaluate and implement the appropriate and effective oral hygiene for each individual client'.

'Poor oral hygiene is probably the most significant factor in the development of most oral diseases' (Torrance, 1990). Health promotion in schools and in the media is now encouraging us to have healthy teeth. However many people are still unaware of the benefits of preventive dentistry, a situation which results in decay, gum disease and premature loss of their teeth. This can be a very distressing situation for relatives and patients who are having to come to terms with the disease. Patients may suffer with painful mouths, ulcers, bleeding, infection and changes in the bone structures causing problems with their teeth or dentures. This can all add to impairment of nutrition, which has a large part to play in the healing process after surgery. Depression, speech problems, communication difficulties, body image and decreased social functioning also influence how a patient will cope with this disease.

Henderson (1960) at the International Council of Nurses believes that 'the state of the patient's mouth is one of the best indicators of patient care'. Hallet (1984) also feels that we have assumed that if a patient is alert, then he or she is undertaking some form of oral hygiene and that his or her mouth is satisfactory. This is not always the case, especially after major surgery.

Following oral surgery or major surgery oral hygiene is more difficult to maintain due to pain, swelling, etc. Hygienists, if they are available, have a key role to play in the maintenance of hygiene at this stage, although all nurses who are involved in the care of such patients should also be proficient. The patient should be assisted and encouraged in maintaining a clean mouth the day after surgery by means of mouthwashes (corsodyl, hot salt water), which should be used regularly, especially after meals. Gentle mechanical cleaning with a brush should also be encouraged, as most patients are afraid that the wounds will fall apart if they use one. Gentle, frequent cleaning is the key to success, rather than occasional scrubbing. In most cases a small-headed, multi-tufted, child-size toothbrush with a fluoride toothpaste is appropriate. Interestingly, Harris (1980) found that 'the normally accepted toothbrush was prejudged by several nurses as an unsuitable tool' and generally observed that nurses considered the foam stick to be the most acceptable tool. However, in 1986 Trenter Rothe *et al.* published a survey on patients receiving 4-hourly mouth care, showing that foam sticks were in fact ineffective in removing debris from the mouth although they still remained the most widely used tool.

High standards of oral hygiene should be maintained not only for the duration of treatment and rehabilitation, but for life.

Immediate post-operative care – intensive-care and high-dependency units

9

Christine van der Valk and Michael Perry

Principles of high-dependency care
Intensive monitoring
Pain management
Medication
Skin care
Nutrition
Communication
In conclusion

Patients' needs vary considerably throughout the course of their illness and its treatment. This is particularly the case following major surgery, when they may require intensive management in the immediate post-operative period. Such intensive or high-dependency care will be described in this chapter.

Medically compromised patients who require emergency surgery may also benefit from intensive 'work-up' prior to surgery in order to optimize their general condition. This has led to the concept known as 'progressive patient care' (PPC). The principle underlying PPC is that as the patient's condition changes, nursing and medical care increases or decreases accordingly. Patients are moved from one nursing site to another in order to receive the quality of care necessary to support them. Grouping patients in this way is an efficient way of delivering highly specialized care, as heavily dependent patients consume a lot of resources.

At one end of the spectrum of care is the intensive-care unit (ICU) which provides continuous, invasive monitoring and highly specialized treatment.

At the opposite end is the general ward. Here the emphasis is more on rehabilitation, with less need for close supervision. Between these two extremes is an intermediate level of care, namely the high-dependency unit (HDU) (see Box 9.1). Patients who require observation and the use of equipment that is not normally available on a general ward are described as being 'high dependency'. The HDU can therefore act as a 'staging post' where those patients who do not need to be in an ICU, yet require more attention than is available on a general ward, can be treated.

BOX 9.1 High-dependency unit (HDU)

The HDU has been defined by the Association of Anaesthetists of Great Britain and Ireland as 'an area for patients who require more intensive observation, treatment and nursing care than can normally be provided on a general ward. Such a unit would not normally accept patients requiring mechanical ventilation, but it could manage those requiring invasive monitoring'.

Most patients who have undergone major head and neck surgery are admitted to either a high-dependency unit or an intensive-care unit immediately post-operatively. Because they are nearly always invasively monitored and frequently ventilated, these patients require a qualified nurse in attendance at all times. The NHS Executive, in their *Intensive and High-Dependency Care Data Collection* (NHS Executive, 1997) describe the criteria for such patients. Units providing ventilation and/or major organ support are classified as 'intensive care'. HDUs can provide one-to-one supervision, enabling close monitoring of fluid balance and oxygen delivery. They also provide inotropic and renal support, intravenous pain relief and limited ventilatory support (e.g. CPAP). Oxygenation, fluid management and adequate pain relief are all essential for a speedy recovery. HDUs have significantly reduced the duration of stay on an ICU.

Although available to all specialties, specific patient groups have been shown to derive particular benefit from high-dependency care. These include cases of post-operative trauma, general surgery, orthopaedics, major head and neck surgery and plastic surgery. Indications for HDU care vary between different units. Important considerations include age, pre-existing disease, ASA score (see Chapter 3) and the type of operation performed. From a maxillofacial viewpoint, patients would include those listed in Box 9.2.

Most patients require only a brief period (24–48 h) in a high-dependency unit and most can return to the ward the next day. Following major surgery (usually major cancer resection and reconstruction), patients are often ventilated overnight and are therefore admitted to an intensive-care unit. Once extubated they would then be transferred to a high-dependency unit where they would continue to receive close monitoring unless they were well enough to go directly back to the ward.

BOX 9.2 Maxillofacial criteria for high-dependency care

- Following major surgery for malignancy
- Following surgery for extensive facial fractures, particularly those extending into the cranial base (e.g. Le Fort II, III, naso-ethmoidal fractures)
- These patients often require prolonged anaesthesia, may undergo significant facial or upper airway swelling, or have coexisting medical problems which may potentially deteriorate after surgery (e.g. ischaemic heart disease, chronic obstructive airways disease, associated head injury)
- Potential airway hazards (e.g. following incision and drainage of Ludwig's angina, surgery to the upper pharynx or bimaxillary osteotomy)
- Patients requiring intermaxillary fixation (IMF) immediately post-operatively
- General causes of deterioration in coexisting but unrelated medical conditions

It is important that surgeons continue to be actively involved in the management of their patients in the post-operative period. This should be a 'team effort', working closely with the anaesthetists and ICU/HDU nursing staff. The surgeon who operates on a patient is still responsible for that patient's care and should remain in close contact with their progress even though they may not be back on the ward.

An intensive-care environment is notoriously overstimulating to the patient. There is always noise, light and activity, no matter how much this is minimized to allow the patient to rest. Sleep is the time when maximum body repair occurs, and this needs to be taken into account when planning care.

Principles of high-dependency care

Airway management

Most major cases will have spent several hours on the operating table, and it may be necessary to ventilate them electively overnight in order to allow the patient time to rest. This also permits further stabilization with minimal disturbance. However, there are occasions when overnight ventilation is insufficient. Swelling of the upper airway can be so great that it would be obstructed without the presence of an endotracheal tube. This can take several days to subside. In such circumstances it may be preferable from a medical and nursing perspective for the patient to undergo tracheostomy, usually at the same time as surgery. With a tracheostomy in place the patient will then generally only need ventilation overnight. The reduced need for sedation, paralysing medication and analgesia, together with the effects of longer-term ventilation, need to be weighed against the communication difficulties and complications associated with a tracheostomy.

Tracheostomy

A secure airway in the intra- and early post-operative period is essential for patients undergoing resection of the mandible, floor of the mouth, tongue, palate, pharynx and larynx. Tracheostomy, of which several types exist (cuffed, non-cuffed, fenestrated and speaking valves), has long been used to achieve this objective. Cuffed tracheostomy tubes allow safe administration of a general anaesthetic, and prevent any secretions from entering the lungs. Indications include:

- upper airway obstruction;
- prevention of aspiration of fluids (cuffed tube);
- retention of secretions (access for suctioning);
- respiratory insufficiency (respiratory, cardiac or neurological disease).

This should be an *elective* procedure (emergency surgical airways are discussed in Chapter 10 on maxillofacial emergencies). Through a small incision midway between the cricoid cartilage and suprasternal notch the tissues are separated, keeping to the midline of the neck. Meticulous haemostasis is essential at all times. Often the thyroid isthmus obstructs access to the trachea and needs to be securely ligated and divided. The thyroid is a highly vascular organ and carelessness in doing this can result in profound bleeding post-operatively. Once the anterior part of the trachea has been defined it is opened, the endotracheal tube withdrawn and the tracheostomy tube inserted into the lumen. Several different access openings in the trachea have been described (a verticle slit, cutting a small hole, or the so-called 'Bjork' flap which is U-shaped and remains attached inferiorly). Each has its own merits and the choice should be made by the operating surgeon. Once it is in place the flanges of the tube need to be securely fastened to the patient and the wound closed.

Complications include the following:

- displacement of the tube;
- tube obstruction from secretions or crusting;
- bleeding;
- tracheal stenosis;
- local tissue injury;
- vocal cord paralysis (the recurrent laryngeal nerve runs alongside the trachea);
- emphysema and pneumothorax;
- chest infection;
- difficulty in reintubation.

Access is through a separate wound that does not extend into the neck dissection, thereby reducing the likelihood of contamination by respiratory secretions. Incisions are usually small, so that eventually there is no need for surgical closure of the stomal skin, and cosmesis is acceptable. Spontaneous closure of the stoma usually occurs within a few days.

The use of large-volume, low-pressure cuffs, and the avoidance of over-inflation of the cuff by repeated and accurate measurement of the cuff pressures, are important for preventing cuff-induced tracheal injury and subsequent stenosis at the cuff site.

Although it provides direct access to the lower respiratory tract for suction by bypassing the larynx, many patients find it difficult to produce an 'explosive' cough which is useful for clearing secretions from the lungs. However, they can be taught to expectorate, and physiotherapists encourage 'huffing' using the diaphragm. With a co-operative and well-humidified patient, very little suction is required, and most patients can effectively clear their lungs on their own.

Methods of artificial ventilation

These include the following:

- intermittent positive pressure ventilation;
- intermittent mandatory ventilation;
- synchronized intermittent mandatory ventilation;
- high-frequency positive pressure ventilation;
- high-frequency jet ventilation;
- high-frequency oscillatory ventilation;
- high-frequency false diffuse ventilation.

Whichever route is taken to ventilate, several factors remain constant.

- Patients need to be monitored to ensure that ventilation is effective and safe. This usually includes ECG monitoring, central venous and arterial pressures, and pulse oximetry. The end-tidal CO_2 and O_2 saturation can be recorded breath by breath to give an indication of arterial concentrations. This needs to be confirmed with arterial blood gas analysis.
- Regular monitoring of the ventilator settings is required to ensure that the machine is working accurately, that changes have not been made without the nurse's knowledge, and that the patient's lungs are moving in unison with the ventilator.
- As gaseous exchange in the lungs normally occurs in a moist environment, humidification is an important feature of ventilation and tracheostomy care. Endotracheal and tracheostomy tubes both bypass the normal humidification process which is carried out within the nose. The drier the trachea, the more sticky the secretions will be. This leads to crusting, with increasing risk of airway obstruction.
- The lip or nostril level of any endotracheal tube must also be noted at each shift change in order to ensure that the tube remains correctly positioned.
- Cuff pressures require monitoring at each shift change to ensure that the pressure exerted by the cuff is the minimum required to maintain an air-tight seal. Unnecessarily high pressures can result in trauma, leading to tracheal stenosis.

- Tracheal suction is required in all ventilated patients and in those with tracheostomy. As with any procedure that bypasses the body's natural defence mechanisms, this should always be a sterile procedure and follow hospital protocol with regard to how often and what size catheter is used in relation to the size of the ET/tracheostomy tube. As soon as tracheostomy patients are able to do so, they should be encouraged to expectorate themselves, so reducing the risk of trauma and infection from suction catheters.
- Tracheostomies also require regular cleaning. Any suture sites and the area around the stoma must be kept clean and dry. The tapes that are used to keep the tracheostomy tube in place need to be changed regularly and monitored to ensure that they are not too tight, in order to allow for any swelling. Depending on the type of tracheostomy tube being used, some have inner tubes which permit cleaning on a regular basis e.g. 4- to 6-hourly. The advantage of inner tubes is that they assist in maintaining the patency of the airway.
- Sufficient sedation, analgesia and occasionally paralysing agents are required to permit the ventilator to breathe for the patient without causing distress. The levels of analgesia must take into account the surgery which the patient has undergone. All infusions are monitored hourly to ensure that the levels being administered match those being prescribed. Consideration must be given to how much analgesia and sedation has been administered when planning to take the patient off the ventilator. Some drugs take a great deal longer to wear off than others and enable the patient to breathe adequately unaided.
- Daily X-rays may be required on ventilated patients to detect signs of infection and barotrauma.
- Physiotherapy is provided regularly to both ventilated patients and those with tracheostomies, to ensure good lung expansion and removal of secretions.

When the patient is considered fit to breathe spontaneously, a trial of breathing is usually carried out before extubation. The patient is allowed to breathe spontaneously through a T-piece, which delivers oxygen-enriched, humidified air. Alternatively, continuous positive airway pressure may be utilized. After approximately 30 min, arterial blood gases are analysed, and if the results are satisfactory the tracheal tube can be removed.

Circulatory support

Reconstruction following excision of head and neck cancer can include direct closure, the use of an obturator, a pedicled flap or a free flap (see Chapter 12). Whereas pedicled flaps retain their original blood supply, a free flap needs to be 'plumbed' into the defect. The type of reconstruction chosen has a direct impact on the care required post-operatively. Whilst the risk of swelling is the same with both types, because the pedicled flap remains attached to its blood supply it is much less vulnerable than the free flap, provided that pressure is not applied to the pedicle. The position of the head is important for maintaining the circulation in the pedicle. For free flaps, the circulation is particularly important. In order for the donated tissue to 'bed in', a number of factors need to be taken into account.

- Good blood flow, with an adequate blood pressure, supplying oxygen and nutrients to the flap and with a good venous drainage are essential. Humidified oxygen is provided at a level that will ensure saturated oxygen levels of > 95 per cent. The concentration of haemoglobin (the transporter of oxygen) is also important. This may need replacement following major surgery, but too high a concentration will increase the viscosity of the blood and reduce blood flow. A compromise therefore has to be reached between oxygen-carrying capacity and the reduction in blood flow through the vessels.
- To enhance the circulation, the blood vessels need to be dilated. This requires the patient to be warm. Temperature control becomes an extremely important factor and requires freedom from draughts which might cool the patient. Most pressure-relieving mattresses have heaters included. Items such as 'space blankets' and 'Bair Huggars' help to raise the temperature following surgery. Nicotine, even from a smoky atmosphere, has been observed to cause almost instant shutdown to the circulation in a flap, so must also be avoided.
- Fluid management is one of the major factors in successful flap management. Patients need to maintain a good perfusion through the flap, and to maintain good renal function. However, fluid excess endangers the cardiorespiratory system, particularly in the elderly where renal function is more sluggish. Good fluid management requires good fluid balance.
- The accurate recording of fluids in and out, on an hourly basis, includes noting all infusions, whether they be crystalloid, colloid (including blood products), drug infusions or intermittent intravenous drugs, including the flush fluids for invasive monitoring. Fluids administered enterally (percutaneous endoscopic gastrostomy, PEG, nasogastric tube, or orally) or parenterally (total parenteral nutrition, TPN) must be taken into account. As the patient progresses and is able to tolerate feeding, fluids are titrated. An hourly level of intake is decided upon by medical staff and the intravenous infusion is reduced as the feeding intake increases. On the debit side, include the urinary output, any drainage from vacuum drains, and any gastric drainage. Diarrhoea and profuse sweating can lead to significant fluid losses. These must all be totalled daily, to provide a 24-h balance. Daily weighing of the patient can be helpful when large volumes of fluids are being lost or gained ($1 \, 1 \, H_2O = 1$ kg) A consistently positive or negative balance has a cumulative effect over a period of days, with an effect on major organ function as well as the health of the flap.

Further care of free-flap patients

The circulation to the flap is checked on an hourly basis for colour (similar to the area from which the tissue came), warmth and venous return. Colour is very important because extreme pallor can indicate a poor arterial supply (although many skin flaps are initially white post-operatively), while a congested dark colour suggests poor venous drainage. Doppler probes are used in some units to provide an auditory clue to blood flow. However, Doppler gives no indication of venous drainage.

Flap management includes oral care. The flap must be warm to permit perfusion. The mouth is normally a warm environment provided that the lips are closed. Intra-oral flaps must also be kept moist but not saturated and chronically wet (macerated). Saliva not only keeps the mouth moist, but is also a useful antibacterial agent. Two-hourly mouth care ensures that the area is kept moist and any exudate from the surgery is removed. If the patient is unable to swallow there is a tendency for secretions to accumulate, requiring gentle suction to remove them. Once patients are able to swallow they are often encouraged to take sips of water (depending on local practice – some consultants prefer free-flap patients to remain nil by mouth for up to 1 week). Not only does this intake help to keep the mouth moist, but it also exercises the oral muscles, encourages the reduction of swelling, and benefits patient morale. Vaseline applied to the lips helps to prevent cracking (a most unpleasant and uncomfortable condition).

The external suture lines are cleaned regularly to prevent the accumulation of dried blood. Sterile cotton buds and saline can be used to roll the suture lines gently. Since the sutures used in facial surgery are very fine, the accumulation of dried blood makes it very difficult to remove them, with the risk of retained sutures causing infection. The greater the level of scab formation, the greater the scarring, which is an important factor in facial surgery. Some units apply a sterile ointment following suturing in order to facilitate removal later.

Donor sites need to be observed for swelling and oozing. For example, if a radial forearm flap has been taken, it is important to check the circulation to the fingers.

Intensive monitoring

The purpose of monitoring is to obtain regular or continuous data following major surgery and responses to treatment. This enables early detection of any deterioration. Useful monitoring techniques are shown in Box 9.3, although not all of them may be necessary in any one individual.

BOX 9.3 Useful monitoring techniques

- Central venous pressure (CVP)
- Arterial blood pressure
- Oxygen saturation (pulse oximetry)
- Temperature
- Pulse and cardiac activity (ECG)
- Pulmonary arterial pressure
- Urine output
- Level of awareness
- Haematology, biochemistry and arterial blood gases

Central venous pressure (CVP)

Central venous pressure is a measure of the pressure in the right atrium and great veins. This depends partly on the pumping ability of the heart and the blood volume. CVP monitoring is therefore useful for assessing the blood volume, and gives an indication of cardiac function. The information from a central line is often used with the urinary output to assess whether the patient requires more or less fluid. This is particularly valuable in elderly patients and those with ischaemic heart disease where excess fluid is poorly tolerated. The normal range for CVP is wide (1–12 cmH$_2$0, 0–10 mmHg), and depends on the patient's position and the reference level (usually the mid-axillary line in the supine patient). The 'filling pressure' can rise considerably in severe heart failure or following massive transfusion. Low values can occur when venous return decreases greatly (e.g. following severe haemorrhage). *Changes* in CVP are a better guide than single readings, and the principle of 'fluid challenge' is useful when a reduced intravascular volume is suspected. After measuring the CVP, a fluid bolus of up to 200 ml is given and the CVP is measured soon afterwards. A transient rise of less than 3 mmHg and no clinical improvements suggest that further volume replacement is necessary. Kinks and blockages in the CVP line and administration of fluid via the monitoring line may give artificially high results.

Central access may be gained by either the subclavian, internal jugular or the antecubital fossa (using a long line), the tip of the catheter being placed level with the right atrium. A high filling pressure is desirable in patients following free-flap surgery in order to maximize flap perfusion, but it must be balanced against the risks of inducing heart failure.

Arterial blood pressure

Blood pressure can be measured using a conventional cuff either manually or automatically. However, peripheral arterial cannulation enables continuous monitoring. The cannula also provides access for taking blood samples for

BOX 9.4 Complications of central venous lines

- Pneumothorax (tension pneumothorax in the ventilated patient)
- Bleeding and haematoma
- Air embolism
- Left-sided catheterization is very occasionally complicated by damage to the thoracic duct and chylothorax
- Wound infection
- Catheter infection. Many units change catheters every 5 to 7 days. Lines carrying parenteral nutrition have an even higher risk. These should always be dedicated to this use only and tunnelled through the skin to reduce infection
- Thrombophlebitis of the vein
- Catheter-tip erosion through the right atrium, resulting in pericardial effusion and occasionally tamponade

blood gases, electrolyte management and blood cell count, etc. The pressure wave form on the monitor provides a visual impression of cardiac function. Arterial lines are generally sited in the radial artery, although the brachial, dorsalis pedis and femoral arteries can be used. A mean arterial pressure of 85 mmHg, or maintaining the normal pressure of the patient, helps to ensure good renal and free-flap perfusion.

BOX 9.5 Complications of radial artery catheter

- Bruising and small haematomas are common
- False aneurysm formation and AV fistula
- Arterial thrombosis
- Inadvertent injection of drugs should not occur, but can be devastating and result in the loss of a hand
- Local abscess and cellulitis which, if unrecognized, can lead to septicaemia. Some units change arterial catheters every 4 to 5 days

Both arterial and central lines require an understanding of their management for monitoring to be accurate. A knowledge of complications is also important, as these can be life-threatening when they arise. Strict aseptic technique is required whenever the lines are accessed. The *Royal Marsden Manual* (Mallett and Barley, 1996) provides information relating to these techniques. The tips of all invasive lines should be cultured following removal, as an aid to eliminating potential infection. Although such lines make life easier and reduce disruption to the patient, by definition they are invasive, they bypass the normal protective mechanisms and they should be treated with respect. As soon as the risks associated with invasive monitoring outweigh the benefits they should (with the permission of the medical staff) be removed.

Pulse oximetry

This is a non-invasive method of monitoring the oxygen saturation in capillary blood and heart rate. A probe consisting of a light-emitting diode and receiver is placed on a digit or ear-lobe. Light is emitted in pulses through the soft tissues, and the degree of absorption represents the percentage of haemoglobin saturated with oxygen. However, this does not represent the partial pressure of oxygen in arterial blood, which must be measured by gas analysis. Saturation permits adjustment of inspired oxygen. It provides an indication of whether the lungs are clear, information on how the patient's temperature is affecting oxygen absorption, and whether the lungs are adequately humidified.

ECG

This assesses pulse rate and heart rhythm.

Temperature

This can be measured using a urinary catheter with a temperature probe included. It provides accurate core temperatures, which are very important in reconstructive surgery, as explained above.

Respiration rate

This needs to be recorded as an indication of lung function, effects of analgesia and sedation, etc.

Sedation levels

These are monitored in ventilated patients. The aim is a comfortable patient who is aware, but not fighting the ventilator. The use of sedation scales, e.g. the New Sheffield Sedation Scale, as recommended by Laing (1992), aids such monitoring.

Pain management

Pain control is one aspect of care about which patients are generally apprehensive beforehand. Uncontrolled pain is one of the most wearing and exhausting factors following surgery. Wherever possible, patients are seen by the nurse specializing in pain management before surgery. There are various methods of effective pain control. Correct breathing technique and the movement of limbs post-operatively are also necessary. Whilst this may appear to fall more within the domain of physiotherapy, a patient must be able to breathe deeply and move about in bed, without being in undue pain, for pain relief to be described as adequate. These factors are also important in the reduction of post-operative complications (e.g. chest infection and deep vein thrombosis). If the patient is pain free, he or she will breathe more easily and move more freely.

Initially, intravenous infusions of opiate drugs would be used both to sedate (if ventilated) and to provide analgesia. Some donor sites (e.g. iliac crests) have a local anaesthetic wound port inserted to provide either intermittent or continuous local anaesthetic medication. Generally speaking, patients are also commenced on non-steroidal anti-inflammatory drugs intra-operatively (if no contraindications exist). These have the advantage of reducing swelling as well as providing pain relief, and in so doing reduce the amount of opiates required. As opiates have a respiratory depressant effect, the sooner the dosage is reduced, the sooner the patient will be able to breathe deeply and sit out of bed. These are elements that not only have a medical benefit, but which also raise patient morale. Not many patients who undergo surgery are accustomed to spending all day in bed. The sooner they can be up and about, the quicker their overall recovery will be.

For some patients there is a need to be in control. They cope with pain better and require less analgesia if they are in control of the administration. Patient-controlled analgesia (PCA) is ideal in this situation. With an appropriate prescription, patients cannot overdose, nor do they have to wait for a nurse to provide the analgesia. However, for it to be successful the patient needs to be able to press the button when analgesia is needed. PCA is unsuitable for the ventilated, sedated and drowsy post-operative patient, for whom continuous infusions are more appropriate initially.

In order to monitor the effectiveness of the analgesia, a pain score chart may be used. The design of the chart at the Queen Victoria Hospital has arisen following extensive research into pain management. Accurate pain score management permits the manipulation of the analgesia in order to maximize pain relief while using minimal medication. Each analgesic infusion is monitored. This ensures that the patient is actually receiving the dosage prescribed, and is a way of checking that the equipment is working accurately.

Medication

The mouth is a notoriously dirty site and the major gateway to the body. Together with the degree of immunocompromise that these patients experience, there is great potential for systemic infection. Following lengthy surgery, particularly involving the oral cavity, antibiotics are prescribed intravenously according to local protocols.

On admission to hospital, all patients have a thromboprophylaxis risk assessment completed. All patients who will be undergoing lengthy surgery will be asked to wear anti-embolism stockings. Depending upon other risk factors, they may also be prescribed low-molecular-weight heparin, e.g. Enoxaparin.

With maxillofacial surgery, it is quite common for patients to develop stress-related gastric erosions. With prevention in mind, patients are generally prescribed an H_2-antagonist, e.g. Ranitidine.

Whenever appropriate the patient's usual medication is continued. One of the risk factors for oral lesions is alcohol. High alcohol intake of any description poses several problems. These patients are all at risk of withdrawal post-operatively when their normal alcohol intake is stopped abruptly. Whilst relevant questions will be asked upon admission so that action can be taken, it is rare for a patient to be honest about the level of alcohol normally consumed. Often it is not until after surgery that the problem comes to light.

Skin care

As part of a programme of practice development, the Queen Victoria Hospital researched and established a file on available pressure-relieving mattresses. The Waterlow Scale (Waterlow, 1995) was used to identify the level of risk. On admission to hospital all patients have their Waterlow score assessed to ensure that a suitable mattress will be available on leaving the operating theatre. As patients may spend an average of 6 h on the operating table, and often have underlying medical problems, their Waterlow score is relatively high. An appropriate pressure-relieving mattress is essential for preventing the development of pressure sores. Following reconstructive surgery and usually ventilation as well, it is not easy to turn patients as frequently as would be necessary (e.g. 2-hourly) on an ordinary hospital mattress. Regular turning under such circumstances requires many nurses and frequent disturbance to the patient.

Each patient has a daily bed bath, with washes as necessary throughout the day. Depending upon which mattress the patient is being nursed on, pressure areas will be checked and washed 4- to 8-hourly. The bed bath includes urinary catheter care and a shave for male patients. As anti-embolic stockings are worn routinely, these need to be taken off at least once a day to check for any signs of pressure.

As soon as patients are aware and able to co-operate, with the help of the physiotherapist they will be asked to breathe deeply to encourage lung expansion, and to move their legs. Good ankle rotation and foot extension and flexion are most effective in encouraging venous return in calf muscles. Until patients are able to move their limbs for themselves, passive limb exercises are essential. However, for patients who are on long-term ventilation and not fully paralysed, it is possible that passive limb exercises can cause damage to the joints, when resistance is encountered.

Depending on the specific surgery, and usually after any invasive monitoring has been removed, most patients are sat out of bed in a chair as soon as possible. This may be for as short a period as 5 minutes or as long as a few hours, entirely depending on the patient. Patients who have undergone tracheostomy often find that sitting in a chair is the most comfortable position for them. Apart from the obvious medical benefits to the patient of getting out of bed (improved circulation, easier lung expansion, etc.) there is the added benefit to their morale. Sitting out of bed is the first step towards recovery, and the patient feels that they are making progress.

Nutrition

Feeding is an important aspect of the care of any patient. Following major surgery that requires a great deal of healing, nutrition becomes even more vital.

Whilst many patients are comparatively fit on admission, many are undernourished. There are several possible reasons for this. A lesion may well make eating and drinking painful, while the disease process can bring about weight loss. Some patients gain most of their calorific intake from alcohol, leading not only to malnourishment but also to an impaired immune system. These patients are very sensitive to the stressful effects of surgery. Although ideally such patients would be admitted prior to surgery in order to provide supplementary feeding, their urgent need for surgery makes this impractical.

Following major surgery, it is often difficult to eat a normal diet. The favoured method of overcoming this problem in our unit is to insert a gastrostomy tube via an endoscope at the time of surgery. A percutaneous endoscopic gastrostomy (PEG) has many advantages over other methods of feeding. Unlike a fine-bore nasogastric (NG) tube, its position does not need to be checked on X-ray, nor is there the same risk of reflux with the potential for aspiration into the lungs. Water can therefore be commenced within a few hours of surgery. There are fewer physical restrictions on long-term feeding with a PEG than with an NG tube. The other potential form of feeding is total parenteral nutrition, usually via a central line into a major vein. Not only is this a very invasive procedure with much greater potential for sepsis, but it does not utilize the normal gut function. Encouraging normal gut function is important. Apart from the obvious need to commence feeding as soon as possible in order to aid healing, there is the added hazard of delayed feeding. Buckley and MacFie (1997) found that where the gut is failing to function, there is an increased risk of bacterial translocation leading to sepsis.

All patients should be referred to a dietitian pre-operatively. Each patient's needs vary according to the underlying medical condition and whether or not they are being ventilated. An individual feeding regime will be prepared and reviewed on a regular basis.

Communication

All patients who are undergoing maxillofacial surgery have a problem with being able to communicate their needs to those around them, especially following major surgery. So long as air is unable to pass over the vocal cords (e.g. due to ventilation with a cuffed endotracheal tube or some types of tracheostomy), speech is not possible. Following surgery to the tongue or the floor of the mouth it becomes physically difficult to talk until the flaps have bedded in, the swelling has reduced and muscles have been encouraged to work again. The resultant sense of isolation and frustration at being unable to explain the most basic of needs is tremendous.

On a simple level, asking questions that require a 'yes or no' answer, i.e. with a nod or shake of a head or one squeeze of the hand for yes and two squeezes for no, means that the nurse has to be extremely observant, understanding, patient and supportive.

Provision of paper and pencil permits more than a yes or no answer, but some patients are reluctant to use this form of communication, either because they feel that their spelling will let them down, or because they think that their writing will be illegible. It is also possible that they require spectacles which will not fit over dressings. There is also the problem of medication impairing thought processes and the physical act of writing. For patients undergoing tracheostomy, a booklet of signs and symbols is provided to enable better communication with staff and relatives following surgery.

Ideally patients are seen by a speech therapist pre-operatively, and this provides an opportunity for them to ask questions before surgery. Furthermore, all patients undergoing major head and neck surgery are visited by one of our staff pre-operatively, ideally a member of staff who will be on duty when the patient comes out of theatre. We explain what the patient might expect following their operation in terms of lines and equipment, how the surgery will affect the patient's ability to communicate, and how we can help. It proves to be an ideal opportunity for patients to ask questions. These can be both about the impending operation and about matters such as visiting times. It also gives the nursing staff an indication of how the patient is likely to cope. The patient benefits from making contact with the staff and being able to recognize a familiar face after surgery.

Part of the care of these patients involves ensuring that everything which is done for them is explained before it is started. It must be remembered that the patient has to be able to give consent, even if he or she is not actually able to speak. This does not mean that written consent is necessary, but following a description of what is planned and why, the patient's response must be noted. Although acceptance of the explanation can be regarded as consent, there is generally a greater response when the patient means 'no'. For example, a refusal to open the mouth for oral care. Before trying again, the reason for non-compliance must be clarified (is the patient in pain? is the patient tired?). It is all too easy in the intensive/high-dependency environment to be constantly doing something to and for the patient. Rest is necessary even when the patient is ventilated and sedated.

One very important aspect of the care of such patients is the support of family and friends. Patients do not usually live in isolation, but are part of a social group. Recovery is greatly aided by allowing visits by the closest members of the social group. This allows contact with the home environment to be maintained. It is this world that the patient has come from and to which in all probability they will return. However, it must also be borne in mind that visitors can be very tiring. Therefore a balance must be achieved between the work of post-operative care, visitors and rest.

In conclusion

Our ward philosophy is that 'all clients will be treated as individuals: the post-operative phase will be unhurried, pain-free and as comfortable as we can make it'. This applies equally to our high-dependency patients and to our recovery patients. The holistic aspect makes the care of patients who have undergone major surgery a constant challenge and always rewarding.

Maxillofacial emergencies

10

Michael Perry and Christine van der Valk

Airway obstruction
Laryngeal trauma
Urticaria and angioedema
Emergency surgical airways
Retrobulbar haemorrhage (RBH)
Penetrating injuries
Oral and facial infections
Epistaxis
Facial palsy
Sinusitis
Septal haematoma

Maxillofacial 'emergencies', i.e. those conditions requiring *immediate* intervention, often surgical, are generally very uncommon. However, they are often life- or sight-threatening and require prompt diagnosis and treatment if death or serious complications are to be avoided. This chapter describes those emergencies that may present to a maxillofacial unit, and their subsequent management.

In many cases the problem is quite obvious (e.g. profuse haemorrhage), even though the precise cause for it may not be. However, other emergencies require a 'high index of suspicion' (e.g. retrobulbar haemorrhage), particularly when dealing with the drowsy or unconscious patient who cannot be assessed thoroughly. Some conditions (e.g. airway obstruction) may cause unconsciousness via hypoxia, the unconsciousness being mistakenly attributed to some other problem (e.g. alcohol consumption or head injury).

Angioedema and *epiglottitis*, both of which are life-threatening in nature, tend to be seen and managed by physicians, although they must always be considered when one is confronted with non-traumatic airway compromise. *Sinusitis* is not an emergency, but is covered in this chapter since untreated serious complications can develop (cerebral abscess/orbital cellulitis).

BOX 10.1   Maxillofacial emergencies

Maxillofacial emergencies include:
- airway compromise from facial/upper airway trauma;
- retrobulbar haemorrhage (RBH);
- profuse haemorrhage from deep soft tissue injury.

'Urgent' cases (i.e. those requiring treatment within 1–2 h) include:
- severe oral and facial infections;
- epistaxis;
- facial palsy.

Airway obstruction

Partial obstruction is often seen in a drowsy patient lying on their back (e.g. following head injury or consumption of drugs or alcohol). Whilst the patient is supine, the relaxed tongue falls back and obstructs the pharynx. Partial obstruction is accompanied by loud snoring, whereas complete obstruction is silent. Agitation should make one consider hypoxia rather than attributing it to alcohol or drugs.

Fractures of the mandible (usually severe and multiple) can also result in the tongue losing its support and falling back, especially when the patient is lying supine. With such high-impact injuries the patient may also have a head injury and therefore associated drowsiness can aggravate the loss of airway control.

Foreign bodies in the upper aerodigestive tract

Objects in the mouth and nose may be swallowed or inhaled, usually in young children. Following facial trauma airway protection with *control of the cervical spine* is the first priority (see Chapter 11). Foreign bodies must be looked for, especially in cases where the patient has been knocked out or remains drowsy. In all cases, missing teeth, dentures, crowns, etc., *must* be accounted for. This may require radiographs of the chest, neck and occasionally the abdomen. Vomiting in the drowsy patient carries a risk of aspiration which can lead to obstruction and pneumonitis. If vomiting does occur, the patient must be turned on their side whilst still immobilizing the whole spine. Simply turning the head may aggravate a cervical spine injury.

Foreign bodies may lodge in the following regions.

- *Pharynx and oesophagus*. Fishbones commonly wedge in the tonsils or the back of the tongue. Sharp, localized pain on swallowing is highly suggestive of this. Radiographs are not completely reliable as many fishbones are composed of cartilage and will not show up. If easily accessible they can be removed under topical anaesthesia. However, if a fishbone cannot be found, the symptoms may be due to abrasion of the mucosa. In such cases this can be treated with simple throat gargles and the patient instructed to return if the symptoms fail to settle. Examination under anaesthesia may then be necessary.

In elderly patients, food may lodge in the oesophagus causing severe retrosternal discomfort (which may mimic cardiac pain) and dysphagia. If the patient can still swallow fluids, sodium bicarbonate can be tried and the patient encouraged to 'belch' the bolus back up. If this does not work, removal using a rigid oesophagoscope will be necessary. Obstruction in the elderly should always raise the suspicion of a stricture (possibly malignant), and further investigations may be necessary.

- *Larynx*. Foreign bodies in the larynx can cause severe airway obstruction with respiratory distress, stridor, cyanosis and respiratory arrest. Immediate attention (which may include the Heimlich manoeuvre) is required, but if this is unsuccessful and the patient is *in extremis*, a surgical airway will be required.
- *Tracheobronchial tree*. Here foreign bodies tend to lodge in the right main bronchus, and the patient will present with shortness of breath, coughing or wheezing. If the foreign body is not removed this will lead to collapse and consolidation of the associated lung. Removal under general anaesthesia using a rigid bronchoscope is necessary.

Laryngeal trauma

The larynx is a semi-rigid structure consisting of a horseshoe-shaped hyoid bone and a collection of small cartilages connected by fibrous tissue. It contains the vocal cords, 'supraglottic' and 'subglottic' spaces. The 'paraglottic' space lies between the lining mucosa and the cartilages. This space is potentially very distensible as a result of bleeding and oedema. The cricoid cartilage lies below the larynx and is the only complete ring in the respiratory tract.

Airflow through a tube varies according to Poiseuille's law (flow = $\pi pr^4/8ln$), where p is the pressure of air, r is the radius of the tube, l is its length and n is the coefficient of viscosity. Small changes in the radius (e.g. from swelling/oedema) can therefore have large effects on the flow of air through the larynx. This is important at the vocal cords – the narrowest part of the upper airway – where the mucosa can swell considerably.

Common causes of injury include the following.

1 Blunt causes:
   - road traffic accidents;
   - sports (e.g. martial arts and racket sports);
   - assaults.
2 Penetrating causes:
   - knife wounds;
   - attempted suicide.

3 Thermal causes:
- inhalation of smoke, hot air or steam.

Types of injury

These include the following.

- Oedema or haemorrhage, which occur particularly after thermal inhalation with rapid reductions in airflow. Early intubation is often necessary.
- Fractured larynx. In young patients, the larynx is elastic and flexes rather than fractures. Blunt injuries tend to bend and displace the larynx, which springs back to its normal position. However, the epiglottis may become avulsed. In older patients the cartilages become calcified and fracture/displacement may occur.
- The trachea can be avulsed from the cricoid cartilage. Displacement is usually rapidly fatal. However, if it springs back, the airway can be maintained but may be displaced subsequently.
- Surgical emphysema of the neck and face may be seen after penetrating or blast injuries.

BOX 10.2   Clinical features

- Dyspnoea/stridor
- Pain/tenderness
- Hoarse voice
- Dysphagia
- Surgical emphysema
- Displacement of the larynx/loss of 'Adam's apple'

Management

In minor laryngeal injuries, humidified oxygen-enriched air and steroids may be required. In severe injuries the airway must be secured by either intubation or tracheostomy (after intubation). Indications for surgery include the following:

- tracheal injuries;
- laryngeal displacment;
- excessive swelling of the laryngeal soft tissues;
- surgical emphysema.

Urticaria and angioedema

These are hypersensitivity conditions which affect up to 15 per cent of the population at some time. Urticaria affects the skin with transient, oedematous, itchy swellings. Angioedema is similar but involves the subcutaneous tissues and mucous membranes, especially around the face. In the rare syndrome of hereditary angioedema, the respiratory tract may be affected, resulting in stridor, which can be fatal. Episodes may be precipitated by drugs, insect stings, specific foods, animals or pollens, or by cold, heat, sunlight, direct pressure, water, vibration or exercise. Viruses and parasites are common precipitants in children. Angioedema can be diagnosed by showing the specific defect of complement C1 esterase inhibitor in the blood.

Treatment

Antihistamines and steroids are the usual treatment for both acute and chronic angioedema. Potential airway obstruction requires immediate intermuscular adrenalin, repeated if necessary and followed by an antihistamine. A surgical airway may be necessary. Patients who have had such an episode should be given adrenalin with clear instructions and a demonstration of how to inject themselves. In hereditary angioedema, donor serum C1 esterase inhibitor concentrate is required. Patients may also be treated prophylactically with Stanasol or Danosol, which raise serum levels of C1 esterase. Tranexamic acid is a less effective alternative.

Emergency surgical airways

In less urgent cases an airway can usually be secured by other means. This depends on the particular circumstances, and includes the use of:

- suction;
- tongue suture;
- chin lift/jaw thrust;
- nasopharyngeal/oropharyngeal airway;
- nasotracheal/orotracheal intubation;
- cricothyroidotomy;
- tracheostomy.

The choice of method depends on:

- the type of obstruction;
- urgency of airway;
- conscious level;
- presence or suspicion of cervical spine injury;
- the experience and skills of the clinician.

Indications for urgent surgical airways include the following:

- actual or potential obstruction;
- laryngeal fractures;
- upper tracheal injury (if unable to intubate).

In all cases supplemental inspired oxygen is necessary.

Most authorites generally agree that the most appropriate *emergency* surgical airway for upper airway obstruction is through the cricothyroid membrane, rather than a tracheostomy. If time allows, a stab incision is made through which a small cuffed tracheostomy or endotracheal tube is passed. Formal tracheostomy takes longer to perform, is more difficult and has potentially more serious complications (see Chapter 9). However, fractures of the larynx may make cricothyroidotomy impossible. In *extreme* conditions, access can be established by passing a brown or grey venflon through the cricothyroid membrane. This can then be connected to oxygen via a Y-shaped cannula, but it is only a temporary measure.

Retrobulbar haemorrhage (RBH)

Bleeding and gross swelling behind the eye may occur after trauma or surgery to the eye or orbit. This is usually seen after retrobulbar injections, fractures of the zygomaticomaxillary complex or the treatment of these fractures. Sight-threatening RBH is rare, with a reported incidence of around 0.3 per cent. It commonly occurs within a few hours of the injury, although cases presenting up to 5 days after injury have been reported.

The orbit is effectivly a rigid, closed 'box', with the globe forming one of its walls. Any swelling will therefore be resisted by the bony walls, and as the pressure behind the eye increases, the eye is pushed forward.

BOX 10.3   Clinical features

- Bulging of the eye
- Progressive pain
- Progressive limitation of eye movement
- Deterioration in vision – *blindness*
- The pupil becomes fixed and dilated
- The globe becomes hard and stony on palpation

Blindness is believed to occur as a result of spasm of the optic and retinal blood supply.

Retrobulbar haemorrhage requires immediate surgical decompression if the eyesight is to be saved. This is achieved through an infra-orbital or lateral eyebrow incision, with blunt dissection passing below and behind the globe to allow drainage. Care must be taken not to injure the optic nerve during this procedure. Following evacuation of the haematoma, a drain is placed to allow escape of further blood and oedema fluid.

When unavoidable delays in surgery occur, short-term measures include the following:

- high-dose IV steroid (1–3 mg/kg stat);
- acetazolamide 250/500 mg IV stat;
- mannitol 100 ml 20 per cent infusion (doses for standard 70 kg adult without medical contraindications);
- lateral canthotomy and cantholysis.

However, drugs take several hours to become fully effective, by which time the patient must be in theatre. A lateral canthotomy (division of the lateral canthus – one of the supporting liagaments attaching the eyelids to the orbital rim) can be performed under local anaesthesia. This provides a little 'breathing space' by allowing the eye to 'pop' forward, reducing the pressure in the orbit. This is also only a temporary measure and should not delay surgery.

Post-operatively, the patient is nursed upright, given effective analgesia, and frequent eye observations are continued should re-collection of blood/fluid occur. Opiates should be avoided as they affect pupillary measurements, and an eye-patch should not be used as this may conceal further deterioration.

Penetrating injuries

These are often very dramatic in appearance, but in many cases they may miss vital structures. Penetrating injuries *deep to the platysma* muscle should not be explored under local anaesthesia in a casualty setting. Irrespective of how dramatic the appearance may be, all penetrating foreign bodies should be left *in situ* until the patient is anaesthetized and has secure intravenous access. Surgical removal can then be undertaken in an operating theatre. Antibiotics and tetanus prophylaxis must be considered.

Oral and facial infections

The following infections may be regarded as potentially life-threatening.

Quinsy (peritonsillar abscess)

This is not acute tonsillitis but infection which has spread into the adjacent tissues, developing into an abscess. Clinically, the patient becomes unwell and pyrexic. They may be dehydrated secondary to dysphagia and limitation of mouth-opening from muscle spasm (trismus). Patients complain of severe unilateral pain, which may be referred to the ear. The tonsil is grossly swollen and inflamed, with swelling extending into the soft palate pushing the uvula to the opposite side. If untreated, rapid spread into the retropharyngeal tissues and parapharyngeal space and septicaemia can occur. Management involves incision and drainage, which can often be carried out under topical anaesthesia. This needs to be accompanied by systemic antibiotics.

Ludwig's angina

Infection arising in the submandibular or submental triangle (usually dental in origin) may quickly spread to involve both sides – effectively the whole of the floor of the mouth. The patient rapidly becomes unwell and pyrexial with gross, tense swelling of the floor of the mouth, which lifts up the tongue. Dysphagia is marked, and they quickly become dehydrated. Failure to treat this condition will ultimately lead to further spread of infection into the para-pharyngeal spaces and airway obstruction. Swelling is not always due to abscess formation, but nevertheless this condition requires urgent incision and drainage to decompress the tense tissues. Intravenous fluids and antibiotics are also required.

Untreated dental infections may lead to abscess formation in various tissue spaces. Most commonly these include submasseteric, submandibular, submental and buccal spaces. All abscesses should be incised and drained as soon as possible, and should not be left until the following day.

Skin infections – cavernous sinus thrombosis

Skin infections around the centre of the face can be potentially serious. Here the venous drainage flows in two directions, into the internal jugular vein or retrogradely into the cavernous sinus in the brain. Retrograde spread of bacteria can lead to thrombosis in the sinus, which is a severe and life-threatening neurosurgical complication. For this reason, any abscess in this region should be incised and drained. 'Spots' should not be squeezed.

Epistaxis

Epistaxis (nosebleed) is common, being reported in up to 10 per cent of the general population at some time. Most cases occur in children, young adults and those over around 55 years of age. In some cases epistaxis may be associated with an underlying condition (e.g. trauma, bleeding disorders, telangiectasia and tumours), and for this reason recurrent epistaxis may need further investigations. Many patients develop spontaneous bleeding or bleeding after trauma, which in most cases settles quickly in response to simple first-aid measures. However, major epistaxis requires prompt treatment, depending on the degree of blood loss and the general condition of the patient.

Bleeding usually occurs from the anterior nasal septum (Little's area), which can be simply controlled by cauterization or pinching the nose. Particularly in the elderly, it may also arise from the spheno-ethmoidal recess, which is higher and further back in the nasal cavity and less easy to reach. Haemorrhage from this region cannot be stopped by compression.

Epistaxis associated with mid-facial trauma can be extremely difficult to manage. It is essential that bleeding is kept under control, but it must be remembered that some fractures may involve the anterior cranial fossa and communicate with the cerebrospinal fluid. Here there is a risk of introducing infection, or of perforating the fragile skull base when placing nasal packs. Whether packing should be undertaken depends on the severity of the facial injuries, the severity of the blood loss and the patient's general condition.

Recurrent or prolonged bleeding may indicate an underlying cause. Such causes include:

- vascular malformations (e.g. hereditary haemorrhagic telangiectasia);
- tumours (e.g. nasal carcinomas, lymphomas, etc.);
- bleeding disorders (idiopathic thrombocytopenia purpura, leukaemia, haemophilia, von Willebrand's disease);
- drugs (particularly anticoagulants);
- hypertension.

Management

Minor bleeds usually resolve on their own, or require only simple first-aid measures (sitting forward and pinching the nose for at least 20 min). If this fails, the vestibule and septum should be examined for bleeding points. These may be cauterized using silver nitrate sticks or needle diathermy under topical anaesthesia. Cocaine paste causes vasoconstriction and helps to control bleeding, but care is needed in its use as too much is toxic. Xylocaine spray can be used instead. Where the bleeding source cannot be seen, the nose can be packed using ribbon gauze impregnated with vaseline or bismuth iodoform paraffin paste (BIPP). More secure packing involves using a soft foley catheter, which is inserted (deflated) through the nose until it is visible at the back of the throat. The balloon is then inflated and gentle traction applied, 'wedging' the balloon between the soft palate and nasopharynx. Ribbon gauze can then be packed anteriorly. Simpler alternatives include commercially available nasal 'tampons'. Packs are generally retained for around 48 h following control of haemorrhage. Antibiotics may be required.

Patients should have their pulse and blood pressure checked, and if bleeding has been severe they should be investigated for bleeding disorders. Elderly patients in particular are affected more by blood loss and may develop postural hypotension or syncope. Occasionally intravenous fluids may be required. Patients who have had major nose bleeds should be admitted for observation, bed rest, pain relief and IV fluids. Following trauma, although they are technically compound fractures, nasal fractures associated with epistaxis do not generally require antibiotic cover.

In rare instances where there is torrential haemorrhage which cannot be controlled by packing, ligation of the external carotid artery and anterior ethmoidal artery may be necessary. The anterior ethmoidal artery passes through the orbit and is exposed via a transorbital approach. This is a 'last ditch' attempt and may be required in cases of continuing major bleeding that are resistant to all other treatments.

Facial palsy

Causes of unilateral facial weakness that are commonly seen in maxillofacial practice include the following:

- head injury;
- herpes zoster infection (shingles);
- Bell's palsy;
- multiple sclerosis;
- parotid/intracranial tumours.

It is important to determine the cause accurately, as the treatments for each of these are completely different.

Head injury

Facial weakness following a head injury usually indicates a fracture involving the temporal bone. Diagnosis is usually clinical with a history of significant trauma. In addition there may be:

- bleeding from the ear;
- haemotympanum (blood visible behind the ear-drum);
- vertigo;
- nystagmus;
- deafness.

Herpes zoster infection (Ramsey–Hunt syndrome)

This is a viral infection, usually chicken-pox, affecting the geniculate ganglion. In addition to facial weakness, vesicles are visible on the ear canal, pharynx and face. Management requires the use of systemic antiviral agents (acyclovir).

Bell's palsy

Idiopathic facial palsy (Bell's palsy) should be a 'diagnosis of exclusion'. All other causes must be eliminated clinically or following investigations. Thorough examination of the head and neck, especially the cranial nerves, is essential before the diagnosis can be made with any degree of confidence. High-dose intravenous steroids may be of use, although this treatment is controversial and if the diagnosis is wrong (e.g. Herpes zoster) will lead to rapid spread and deterioration in the patient. The prognosis for Bell's palsy is generally good.

Parotid tumours (see Chapter 13)

Ocular complications

Inability to close the eyelid in severe weakness may lead to drying of the conjunctiva and corneal damage. In the first instance this may be managed by artificial tears, taping the upper lid down and applying an eye-patch. If no signs of improvement are seen, a lateral tarsorrhaphy may be carried out as an intermediate measure. This involves suturing the lateral aspects of both upper and lower eyelids together to improve tear retention.

Sinusitis

Acute sinusitis

This is common after 'colds' where inflammation and mucous secretion by the sinus mucosa block the osteum and paralyse the cilia. Stagnant secretions can then become infected. The maxillary sinus is usually affected. Acute frontal sinusitis, although less common, is more likely to cause serious complications. The ethmoidal sinuses, between the orbits, have a thin lateral wall, so inflammation can spread laterally resulting in orbital cellulitis. This is potentially sight- and life-threatening. Children suffer from acute sinusitis less often than adults because the sinuses are not fully developed, but when they do have this condition they may present with cellulitis of the eyelids or, more rarely, of the orbit. This requires intravenous antibiotics and, if an abscess is present, surgical drainage.

Diagnosis is usually clinical, with symptoms of malaise, headache, low-grade fever, facial pain or discomfort (worse later in the day and on stooping), nasal obstruction, post-nasal drip and mucopurulent nasal discharge.

Treatment

Acute sinusitis often resolves spontaneously within several weeks. Antibiotics may be required if the symptoms are severe or prolonged. Vasoconstrictor drops may aid drainage but can cause rebound swelling if they are given for longer than 10 days. Simple steam inhalations are often sufficient to relieve symptoms. Surgery is not required for simple acute sinusitis. However, antral lavage may be required if there is severe pain or systemic symptoms.

Chronic sinusitis

This may require a simple antrostomy (drainage procedure) performed through the inferior or middle meatus within the nose. Radical antrostomy through the canine fossa may be necessary when simple drainage fails. This provides good access and allows removal of the mucosa and treatment of any associated dental problems.

Septal haematoma

Septal haematomas are seen following nasal injuries and require urgent treatment. Failure to provide this can result in necrosis of the septum which, if severe, leads to noisy breathing ('whistle deformity') and nasal deformity. Haematomas may be simply aspirated, but may require open drainage under local anaesthesia.

Maxillofacial trauma

Krys Peel and Michael Perry

This chapter describes the assessment and management of facial fractures (see also Chapter 4). It is important to remember that in most cases treatment can wait and other injuries, particularly of the head and neck, must take priority.

Initial assessment

Minor injuries to the face are very common in the UK, whereas major facial trauma is less frequently seen. This is partly due to seat-belt and drink-driving legislation, which has significantly reduced the number of deaths from road traffic accidents (RTAs). However, in some cases patients who would previously have died at the scene as a result of head injuries now survive with serious facial injuries. Sporting injuries and assaults account for the vast majority of the remaining injuries.

In assessing patients with multiple injuries the initial priority is to determine whether any life-threatening injuries exist and to deal with them first. The advanced trauma life support system (ATLS) is one such approach in which, during a 'primary survey', life-threatening injuries are identified and treated as they are found. Most maxillofacial injuries can wait for treatment, and only occasionally do they require immediate management (see Chapter 10).

Once the 'primary survey' and 'resuscitation' phases have been completed, attention can then be focused on the maxillofacial region. In this context the following points can be made.

1 *Facial injuries.* These can put the airway at risk, particularly when consciousness is reduced by associated head injury, alcohol or drugs. Early identification and immediate action are essential if brain damage is to be avoided. The airway should be cleared of debris, saliva, broken teeth or dentures, either manually or by suction, and when possible the patient should be nursed upright to maintain patency and reduce the effects of swelling (unless other injuries contraindicate this position; see below). The chin lift or jaw thrust help to improve the airway initially in obtunded patients and, where necessary, an oral or nasopharyngeal airway may be placed. If the patient is unconscious and unable to maintain their airway with these measures, a definitive airway is indicated. This usually requires intubation, but if this is not possible (e.g. in shotgun injuries), a surgical airway may be required. Long-term security of the airway can be achieved by tracheostomy. However, this should not be carried out as an emergency procedure.

2 *Cervical spine injuries. All patients with multiple injuries and particularly those with a significant injury above the clavicle should be assumed to have an injury to the cervical spine until it is proven otherwise.* A high index of suspicion is essential. Until this has been excluded, the whole spine should be immobilized. Adequate cervical spine immobilization requires a hard cervical collar supported by sandbags and tape.

3 *Bleeding.* With the exception of gunshot wounds and lacerated major vessels, *isolated* facial injuries rarely bleed enough to cause shock. If shock is present, other causes must be found. Bleeding can usually be controlled by local pressure dressings, and nasal packs can be used for bleeding from the nasal spaces (see Chapter 10).

4 *Head injuries.* Fractures of the anterior cranial fossa have similar clinical features to some upper facial fractures (e.g. naso-orbitalethmoidal), and are often associated with them. These are significant head injuries and should be managed as such initially, with close observation (Glasgow Coma Scale) and CT scanning if indicated (Fig. 11.1). Nasal packs, nasogastric tubes and nasopharyngeal tubes should not be passed.

5 *CSF leaks.* Facial fractures which extend into the skull base (e.g. Le Fort II, Le Fort III, naso-orbitalethmoidal) can tear the dural lining and allow cerebrospinal fluid (CSF) to leak from the nose (rhinorrhoea) (Fig. 11.2). This presents as a heavily bloodstained, persistent watery discharge which trickles down the side of the face. Peripherally the blood clots form two parallel lines, referred to as 'tramlining'. The 'ring test' is helpful for distinguishing between CSF and mucus.

6 *Penetrating neck injuries deep to the platysma muscle.* These should not be explored on the ward or in a casualty department, due to the risk of major haemorrhage.

7 *Swelling develops rapidly.* Assess the eyes early before swelling develops and prevents later assessment.

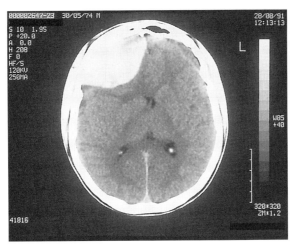

Figure 11.1 Acute extradural haematoma. Head injuries and cervical spine injuries always take precedence over maxillofacial injuries.

8 *Analgesia.* Pain is seldom severe, even following major maxillofacial trauma. The usual complaint is of discomfort due to the swelling. Analgesia may be given as appropriate to the patient's current condition and past medical history, noting any allergies. Strong analgesics, such as opiates, which may depress the level of consciousness or respiration rate should be avoided, since strictly speaking all facial injuries are also 'head injuries'. Mobile fractures, (e.g. of the mandible) can be stabilized temporarily by placing wire loops around the teeth (bridle wire) under local anaesthesia.

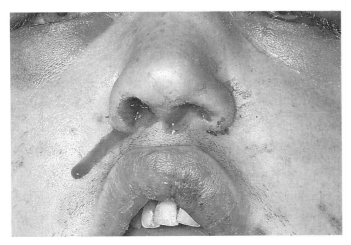

Figure 11.2 Cerobrospinal fluid (CSF) rhinorrhoea. Watery discharge from the nose following a head injury should always be regarded as indicating a CSF leak until proven otherwise.

9 *Post-traumatic symptoms.* These may include nightmares resulting from the trauma, and sleep may be disturbed for some time. Time is usually the best healer for these dreams, but occasionally some patients can be adversely affected for a long time, and in extreme cases counselling may prove beneficial.

The facial skeleton

Many bones make up the facial skeleton. These include:

- the upper third (frontal bone);
- the middle third, between the supra-orbital ridges and the upper teeth (two maxillae, two zygomas, two lacrimal bones, two nasal bones, one vomer and one ethmoid);
- the lower third (mandible).

Some bones, such as the ethmoid and orbital roof, are so thin that on a dry skull light can easily pass through. The remainder vary in thickness but are often quite delicate (nasal, zygoma). The mandible is the strongest of the facial bones.

The face is not solid but contains several 'cavities', including the sinuses, orbits and nasal cavity. Around these the bones form a series of vertical struts or 'buttresses'. Facial bones are very effective at resisting vertically directed forces (e.g. during chewing), but are relatively weak in the horizontal direction (i.e. during most injuries). This results in most of the impact being absorbed by the face, thereby protecting the brain (see section on mid-face fractures). Fractures may be described as simple, comminuted, compound or pathological (where pre-existing bone disease has weakened the bone, e.g. osteoporosis or tumour).

Clinical features

These vary according to specific injuries. Important signs to look for include the following:

- CSF rhinorrhoea or otorrhoea;
- haemotympanum (blood behind the tympanic membrane), which may indicate fractured base of skull or middle-ear injury;
- Battle's sign;
- tears in the external auditory meatus (condylar fractures);
- generalized swelling ('balloon' face), which often indicates severe mid-facial injuries;
- well-demarcated 'Panda' or 'black-eyes' (peri-orbital haematoma), which indicates a fracture involving the orbit. Since the anterior cranial fossa forms the orbital roof, this sign, particularly when bilateral, suggests a skull base fracture;
- trauma to the naso-orbitalethmoidal region (the bridge of the nose, and between the eyes) can separate the inner attachments of the eyelids (medial

canthi). The eyes appear to be too far apart, although it is the medial corners that have become displaced – increased intercanthal distance;

- enophthalmus (sinking back of the eye) and hypoglobus (a drop in the pupillary level) may indicate an orbital 'blowout' fracture or badly displaced fractured zygoma. There may also be limitation of eye movements;
- subconjunctival haemorrhages extending from behind the eye, which suggest a fracture;
- numbness of the face (trigeminal nerve) may suggest a fracture, although a direct blow to the nerve itself may be the cause;
- bruising of the palate or under the tongue indicates underlying fractures;
- inability to bite normally.

Facial bones and the surrounding soft tissues are highly vascular. Thus the initial appearance of the patient is one of blood, teeth and saliva 'everywhere' and can be quite distressing to witness. However, it should be remembered that although facial injuries can appear alarming, an isolated injury in a conscious patient is rarely life-threatening (Fig. 11.1). Swelling around the site of injury is normally at its worst 48 h post-injury. Even if the patient is nursed upright, severe swelling following facial trauma can be upsetting to witness. It should be stressed that the swelling appears very quickly following trauma, but also subsides very quickly once it has 'peaked' at 48 h. Complete resolution can take a few weeks, but most of the swelling reduces within 7–10 days.

Timing of surgery

Although most maxillofacial injuries can wait, late repair (once the fractures have united) is extremely difficult. Early treatment (within 5–10 days) gives the best results, but immediate surgery may be carried out for life-threatening injuries or if the patient is going to theatre for some other reason. The patient and family will be advised by the surgeon that, depending on the nature of the injury, it may not be possible to restore the face totally to its pre-injury state. By delaying surgery for several days:

- observation for head or 'missed' injuries is possible;
- further medical details can be obtained;
- pre-injury photographs may help in the assessment;
- facial swelling will settle, enabling more detailed examination;
- quality radiographs can be obtained (e.g. face, teeth);
- further investigations can be performed (e.g. CT scan, study models, vitality testing);
- aids to surgery can be fabricated (e.g. custom-made arch bars, gunnings splint).

Treatment principles

These include the following:

- debridement – thoroughly clean any open wounds;
- reduce the fracture – open/closed;
- fix the fracture – IMF/internal/external;
- restore function (rehabilitation);
- early and late care of soft tissues (see Chapter 4).

DEBRIDEMENT (see Chapter 4)

All wounds need to be thoroughly cleaned as soon as possible. Skin wounds need to be cleaned gently and prevented from drying out with antiseptic-soaked swabs. Remember tetanus prophylaxis. Oral hygiene is particularly important with fractures of the mandible and maxilla, as these often communicate with the oral cavity which, due to pain, is difficult for the patient to keep clean. Regular use of antiseptic mouthwashes (e.g. corsodyl) and hot salt-water mouthwashes is beneficial. In theatre, dead tissue is excised but this is kept to a minimum. The wounds are thoroughly irrigated and, if grit is ingrained, they are scrubbed.

OPEN REDUCTION AND INTERNAL FIXATION (ORIF)

This involves exposing and reducing the fracture(s) under direct vision, which enables more precise reduction than 'closed' methods. Whenever possible (e.g. in mandible, maxilla and some zygomatic fractures) this is done via the mouth in order to avoid skin incisions. However, if there are overlying lacerations these may be used instead. Although saliva contains numerous organisms, with good surgical technique and appropriate use of antibiotics post-operative infection is surprisingly uncommon. This is in part due to the excellent blood supply to the face and the capacity to fight infection. Methods of fixation include wiring, pins and plates and screws. Plates may be adaptional plates (semi-rigid), compression plates (rigid) or mesh. A 'lag-screw' technique may be possible for some overlapping fragments.

There have recently been developments in the use of 'biodegradable' materials in fracture fixation. These include polylactide (PLA), polyglycolic acid (PGA), and their copolymers, which are said to degrade to carbon dioxide and water. Fractures may therefore be fixed using these materials, which remain in place until the fracture has healed, and subsequently completely disappear. This would reduce the likelihood of infection and the need for subsequent plate removal. At present this approach is still experimental, although encouraging results are being published.

RIGID INTERNAL FIXATION (MANDIBLE ONLY)

This uses heavy metal plates and screws to immobilize fractures *rigidly*. The strength of the plate enables immediate return of function, and the patient can eat soon afterwards. Intermaxillary fixation is not needed. However, this technique risks damaging the inferior dental nerve or teeth. Plates may become infected and the wound may break down.

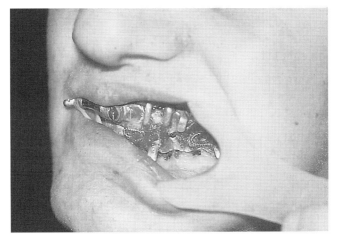

Figure 11.3 Intermaxillary fixation. Although it is very effective, with the advent of miniplates and open reduction and internal fixation (ORIF) of fractures, this method of treatment is now required less often.

INTERMAXILLARY FIXATION (IMF)

This form of immobilization uses the patient's bite to reduce and stabilize fractures, which means that it can only be used for those fragments that are firmly attached to healthy teeth (usually the mandible or dento-alveolar fractures) (Fig. 11.3). It is also commonly used in the treatment of condylar fractures. Fracture reduction is 'blind' and often non-precise. Methods include eyelet wiring, arch bars, cast-cap silver splints and gunning splints (edentulous fractures). Caution is needed with post-operative airway problems, COAD, head injury, epileptics, patients who are likely to vomit, and those with psychiatric disorders. IMF needs to be in place for 2 to 3 weeks and patients may lose weight as a result.

EXTERNAL FIXATION

This involves inserting rigid pins into the bones via the skin, which are then joined by universal joints and connecting rods or splints (Fig. 11.4). This method is particularly useful where tissue has been lost – 'discontinuity defects' (e.g. gunshot injuries), and in infected, severely comminuted and pathological fractures. Fixation can be applied rapidly. However, reduction is 'blind', and the pins may damage the inferior dental nerve or teeth. Patient activity is also restricted, and the pin sites may become infected and scarred.

Antibiotics, steroids and tetanus prophylaxis

Protocols vary between different units. Antibiotics are usually given for fractures which are exposed to saliva or the environment (compound or

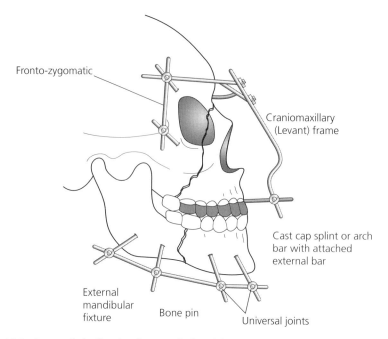

Fronto-zygomatic

Craniomaxillary
(Levant) frame

Cast cap splint or arch
bar with attached
external bar

External
mandibular
fixture

Bone pin

Universal joints

Figure 11.4 External pin fixation for maxillofacial fractures.

'open'). A combination of a penicillin and metronidazole is one suitable choice. The use of prophylactic antibiotics in CSF leakage is controversial, and the opinion of a neurosurgeon should be sought. Tetanus prophylaxis should be considered, especially in 'mucky' wounds, which should be thoroughly cleaned as soon as possible. Steroids (e.g. dexamethasone) are often given to reduce facial swelling.

Fractures of the mandible

The mandible is a 'V'-shaped tubular bone consisting of an outer dense 'cortical' layer enclosing delicate 'trabecular' bone. Through this runs the inferior alveolar nerve. Anatomically it is composed of the symphysis, parasymphysis, body, angle, ramus, coronoid and condyle. The relative frequencies of fractures of these sites are as follows (Fig. 11.5):

- condylar neck   35 per cent;
- angle   20 per cent;
- body   20 per cent;
- parasymphysis   13 per cent;
- symphysis   11 per cent;
- coronoid   1 per cent.

Multiple fractures are more common than isolated fractures.

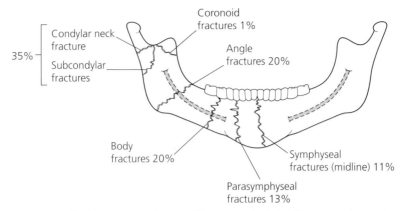

Figure 11.5 Mandibular fractures described by anatomical site. Note that the angle and body fractures involve the inferior alveolar neurovascular canal.

The mandible is strong in front but progressively weakens towards the condyles. Teeth, particularly the long-rooted canine and partially erupted wisdom teeth, tend to weaken the bone. When teeth are present, adjacent fractures usually extend into a socket and may fracture the tooth roots. The socket provides access to the fracture site for bacteria in the saliva, and the site is therefore termed 'open' (compound). This increases the risk of infection. In the edentulous mandible the absence of teeth means that the mucoperiosteal lining tends to remain intact. These fractures are therefore termed 'closed', and there is less risk of infection. However, following tooth loss, localized bone resorption occurs which weakens the bone, and fractures of the edentulous mandible can occur after relatively minor trauma.

Common clinical features include the following:

- pain, swelling and tenderness;
- sublingual haematoma;
- movement and crepitus at the fracture site;
- abnormal 'bite' and step deformity of teeth/lower border;
- numbness of the lower lip (inferior dental nerve);
- bleeding from the ear – tearing of the ear canal may be seen with condylar fractures.

A patient presenting with a fractured jaw may be reluctant to open their mouth for examination. However, they should be encouraged to do so, in order to allow a complete but gentle examination by the medical staff.

Treatment

This aims to restore the patient's bite (occlusion) and appearance, with an early return of chewing, movement and speech. Not all fractures of the mandible require surgery. Surgery may not be required if there is:

- minimal displacement of a stable fracture with minimal mobility;
- normal biting together by the patient;
- no infection;
- good patient co-operation and follow-up.

In these cases treatment consists of a soft diet, analgesics, antibiotics (if compound) and regular follow-up to detect early displacement. For other fractures, or where this fails, the options include:

- intermaxillary fixation (IMF) for 4–6 weeks;
- open reduction internal fixation (ORIF) with wires (plus IMF);
- ORIF using lag screws or plates;
- closed reduction with external fixation.

IMF can be applied by placing wire loops around the upper and lower teeth, or cementing brackets on to healthy teeth which are then used to fix the bite together. This has traditionally been used for many years, and is known to give satisfactory results. In many units in the UK fixation is now achieved using 'miniplates' that are inserted via the mouth. Often IMF is not needed, which is particularly helpful in epileptics, alcoholics, etc. If anatomical reduction is not achieved, a short period of elastic IMF (2–3 weeks) may be used to guide the bite into a better position.

FRACTURES INVOLVING TEETH

If possible, teeth are retained, particularly in front where they can be seen. However, removal may be necessary if a tooth is diseased, damaged beyond repair or interfering with fracture reduction, but removal can occasionally destabilize fracture, making reduction difficult.

Edentulous mandibular fractures

Fractures of the edentulous mandible may be treated using the patient's dentures (if a good fit) or customized 'gunning splints' (essentially modified dentures). These are wired to the upper and lower jaws and then fixed together. In selected cases open reduction and internal fixation using miniplates may be performed. This is preferable if the patient has serious chest disease.

In some units, fractures of severely atrophic mandibles (less than 1 cm thick) are splinted using the patient's own rib. The fracture is sandwiched between a 'split' rib and secured using wire or screws. The rib acts as both a 'miniplate' and a bone graft to encourage healing. A local anaesthetic infusion into the chest wound post-operatively aids early mobilization and adequate ventilation, and minimizes the likelihood of chest infection.

Treatment of condylar fractures

Temporomandibular joint pain, and abnormal mandibular growth or ankylosis in children, are sometimes seen with these fractures in the long term.

Where the occlusion is normal these are generally managed with rest, a soft diet and simple analgesics. These are not compound fractures, so antibiotics are not necessary. Regular review is essential in the early stages to ensure that the fracture does not 'slip' and derange the bite. However, fractures with an associated malocclusion need to be reduced. This is often achieved using rigid or elastic IMF for 2–3 weeks only to avoid ankylosis. Post-operatively, patients fixed in IMF need close monitoring of their airway during recovery from the anaesthetic. This usually requires an overnight stay on an ICU or HDU. Following IMF, jaw movements and physiotherapy are required.

Bilateral condylar fractures may be managed similarly. However, these fractures must be kept under close review until they have healed. 'Telescoping' of the condyles can lead to the occlusion being propped open at the front – an anterior open bite. This would require surgical correction at a later date.

Alternatively, and where IMF is contraindicated (see above), fractures may be exposed and fixed using miniplates, wires or screws. The skin incision is placed just behind the angle of the jaw below the ear. This procedure carries a small risk of facial nerve injury.

Fractures in children

Similar treatment principles apply, and early jaw movements are desirable. If plating is necessary, care must be taken not to damage the unerupted teeth. 'Microplates' are often used. Long-term follow-up during growth is necessary to detect disturbances of growth.

General points in management

Patients should be nursed upright to maintain patency of the airway, unless other injuries contraindicate this position. Often the patient is reluctant to open their mouth, but oral hygiene is important both pre- and post-operatively, especially after food. A clean mouth not only helps the patient to feel more comfortable, but also reduces the risk of infection. The use of a soft toothbrush and toothpaste can be encouraged, but if this is not possible, regular mouthwashes of corsodyl or difflam may be helpful. If, due to discomfort, the patient is reluctant to moisten their lips, petroleum jelly should be available.

Oral fluids should be encouraged pre-operatively until the patient is to be admitted to theatre. Occasionally an intravenous infusion to maintain hydration may be required in reluctant patients. A fluid-balance chart should be maintained in either case in order to check that there is adequate hydration.

Diet is dependent on the injury and subsequent surgery. Patients usually require a soft diet so that mastication causes minimum discomfort to the fracture site and the plates do not distort. Most patients are able to manage a soft or liquid diet. Nutritional drinks should be encouraged but should not be relied upon completely to provide all of the nutritional requirements. The dietitian is a key member of the multidisciplinary team and should ideally visit the patient both pre-operatively and post-operatively. A high-calorie, high-protein diet is desirable. The dietitian can assess the patient's nutritional requirements and give advice on diet, which the patient can follow at home.

Currently it is unusual for a patient to require rigid IMF. If it is to be applied, the patient should be warned pre-operatively about having their jaws wired together. They are less likely to panic when they wake up and are unable to open their mouth if they are psychologically prepared for this beforehand. It is perfectly possible to breathe via the nose or even through the mouth with the wires *in situ*. In the rare event of the patient vomiting once the wires are *in situ*, he or she should be seated upright and forward, to allow the vomitus to drain between the natural gaps between the teeth. It is rarely necessary to cut the wires.

Dietary intake is obviously more problematic if the jaws are wired together. The dietitian should visit the patient and draw up an individual nutritional assessment plan which they can follow at home. The diet needs to be liquidized, but each meal should consist of freshly prepared foods which have been liquidized, rather than relying on high-energy drinks four times a day. The patient will lose some weight (up to a stone), but once a normal diet has been resumed on removal of the wires at 4–6 weeks, the weight will return. Following ORIF, patients can manage a soft diet but should be discouraged from biting into apples or eating toffee, etc., for up to 6 weeks post-operatively, as this can put unnecessary strain on the repair site.

Oral hygiene is also more difficult, especially after each meal. The outer teeth and wires can be cleaned, using toothpaste and a toothbrush, although care should be taken around each wire. The backs of the teeth can be cleared using the tongue and toothpaste. A proprietary mouthwash can be used, but its continued use may discolour the teeth around the wires. This discoloration is easily removed by the dentist once the wires have been removed. Ensure that the wire is not cutting into the gums or lips. Any sharp pieces can be protected with dental wax. As the patient cannot lick his or her lips, the use of petroleum jelly is encouraged.

In the rare event that the patient is choking and the wires need to be cut, a pair of wire-cutters or extremely sharp scissors should be kept near the patient at all times. Prior to discharge, the patient and relatives should be aware of which wires to cut in an emergency. The patient should also be able to demonstrate that they can perform adequate oral hygiene, and should be advised to avoid contact sports for up to 3 months to allow the repair to mature. Damage to nerves may result in a degree of anaesthesia or paraesthesia which may be permanent. Sensation will usually return over a period of 2–3 months, but the interim numbness can be distressing to the patient, especially if lip function is impaired (e.g. dribbling when drinking or difficulty in kissing).

The patient should be advised to avoid smoky environments that may cause sneezing which, in turn, may put pressure on the repair. Tie wires are sometimes removed at 3–4 weeks and elastic bands placed *in situ* for the remaining 1–2 weeks. This allows the jaw slightly more mobility and helps to reduce stiffness. Alcohol consumption and smoking should be avoided, as they can increase the risk of vomiting.

Complications of mandibular fractures

These include the following:

- infection;
- malocclusion;
- restricted mouth opening;
- delayed union/non-union;
- growth disturbance in children;
- exposure of plates and wires;
- injury to ID nerve.

Dislocated mandible

The mandibular condyle articulates with the base of the skull in the glenoid fossa, forming the temporomandibular joint (TMJ). Displacement from the fossa is termed dislocation of the condyle. This may occur on one or both sides. If a fracture is also present, this is known as a 'fracture dislocation'. Clinically, the patient is unable to close their mouth. If only one side is dislocated, the chin is deviated to the opposite side. Rarely, and following severe injuries, the condyle may be driven up into the skull. If seen early, reduction may be possible under local anaesthetic with or without sedation. However, if the patient has marked muscle spasm it may need to be performed under general anaesthesia. Longstanding dislocation may require open reduction. Fracture dislocation may be treated by IMF or by open reduction and internal fixation of the condylar fracture.

Recurrent dislocation may be treated by:

- IMF;
- injection of 'sclerosant' solutions to produce scarring of the lax capsule;
- capsular plication;
- eminectomy;
- augmentation of the eminence.

Zygomatico-maxillary complex ('cheek-bone') fractures

These fractures are common and are often associated with sporting injuries or assaults. Patients usually present with:

- pain, tenderness and swelling;
- flattening of the cheek;
- numbness of the cheek;
- black eye;

- subconjunctival haemorrhage;
- epistaxis.

In all cases, the fracture passes into the orbit and can therefore affect the eye. The soft tissues around the globe can become trapped, restricting eye movements – the 'blowout fracture' (see section on orbital fractures). Although they are relatively minor injuries, these fractures predispose, albeit rarely, to retrobulbar haemorrhage (see Chapter 11) and severe infection around the eye (orbital cellulitis). It is therefore important that the eye itself is assessed, especially with regard to visual acuity and eye movements. The fracture also involves the maxillary sinus and, following nose blowing or sneezing, air may be blown through the fracture into the overlying soft tissues (surgical emphysema). Involvement of the sinus predisposes to sinusitis.

Minimally displaced fractures are managed conservatively with antibiotics, avoiding nose-blowing, and follow-up. Surgery is indicated where there is:

- facial deformity;
- limitation of eye movements;
- limitation of mouth opening.

Fractures may be reduced using a variety of techniques. A commonly used method is the 'Gillies lift' (Fig. 11.6). This involves introducing an elevator through a skin incision in the temple (within the hairline), and directing it under the zygomatic bone (and arch), which is then elevated while an assistant holds the head. Alternatively, a 'malar hook' may be passed under the zygomatic 'buttress' through the skin. Following reduction, the fracture is assessed for stability. If it is stable, any wounds are closed and a 'forced duction test' is carried out to ensure there is no restriction of eye movements. If the fracture is found to be unstable, this requires fixation (usually ORIF) using plates. These may be used in varying combinations, although in many instances a single buttress plate placed through the mouth is all that is required. Rarely, external pins or transnasal wires may be used to fix the fracture.

The timing of surgery depends on the amount of swelling and other factors, such as associated head and eye injury. A *penetrating* eye injury may contraindicate surgery. Otherwise, reduction is usually carried out either immediately or after about 1 week once the swelling has settled. Surgery is usually performed under general anaesthesia, although in selected cases local anaesthesia with or without sedation can be used. However, in rare instances profound stimulation of the vagus nerve may occur during the 'lift'.

General points in management

On admission, baseline neurological and vital signs are recorded. Specific eye observations are required for all patients presenting with fractures

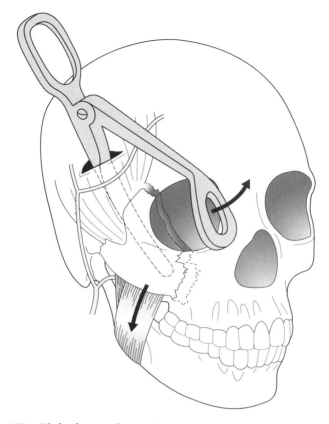

Figure 11.6 Gillies lift for fractured zygoma.

around or involving the orbit both pre- and post-operatively. Eye observations, to include visual acuity, pupil reactivity, pain and proptosis, are performed as the injury indicates. In general, a sliding scale is adopted such as
$1/4$ h × 2 h, $1/2$ h × 2 h, 1 h × 2 h, 2 h × 2 h, although this may vary between
different units. Maintenance 4-hourly eye observations may also be required.
If reduced vision or eye movement is suspected, visual acuity should be
tested. Any deterioration in eye observations must be reported to the medical staff immediately, as it may indicate the development of a retrobulbar
haemorrhage.

Although the side of the fracture is obvious in most cases, this is not always
so, and it is important that the fracture site is marked (by the surgeon)
following surgery. This serves as a reminder to all involved, including the
patient, that pressure over the site must be avoided in order to prevent the
zygoma from redisplacing. The patient should be nursed upright to reduce
swelling and should avoid lying on the affected side. The face often appears
depressed over the fracture site, and the patient usually complains of a black
eye with localized bruising. Immediately post-operatively regular eye observations are continued. Non-steroidal anti-inflammatory drugs (NSAIDs)
and/or dexamethasone may be of benefit in reducing oedema, and some

units prescribe an 'antral regime' (nasal decongestant, menthol inhalations and antibiotics) for about 5 days to prevent sinusitis. Eye care should be performed as required, using warm water or saline. Eyedrops or ointments can be given as prescribed, but the patient should be advised that ointments may blur his or her field of vision. It is important to ensure that swollen eyelids are opened manually on a regular basis. Chloramphenicol ointment may be applied to the conjunctiva and skin incisions to prevent crusting, and chlorhexidine mouthwash aids oral hygiene.

Most patients are fit for discharge on the following day. Eyelid sutures are often removed at 3 days to minimize scarring, and hairline sutures are removed at 7–10 days. Care should be taken with a hairline suture line when washing the patient's hair. A mild shampoo should be used to reduce the risk of scar irritation. A soft diet is encouraged for 2–4 weeks to reduce any discomfort around the fracture site, as chewing may prove uncomfortable. Lost sensation should begin to return at about this time.

The repair needs time to settle, so the patient should be advised to avoid any contact sports for 2–4 weeks. Sneezing, stooping and nose-blowing should be avoided, and the patient should keep off the affected side while sleeping, in order to reduce the risk of dislodging the repair until the final review at 4–6 weeks.

Orbital fractures

These may occur in isolation ('blowout fractures'), but are often associated with zygomatic or nasoethmoidal fractures (Fig. 11.7). Isolated orbital roof fractures are uncommon, but it must be remembered that this is also the delicate anterior cranial fossa, which therefore represents a significant head injury.

Clinical features include the following:

- orbital bruising and swelling;
- subconjunctival haemorrhage and oedema;
- enophthalmus;
- proptosis;
- numbness of the cheek;
- diplopia and restricted eye movements;
- epistaxis.

Early ophthalmic consultation is essential to exclude any eye injury. Management of the eye takes priority over the fracture itself. Very often the eyelids are closed due to painful swelling. However, gentle pressure for a few minutes reduces this sufficiently to allow visual acuity, pupillary size and reaction to be checked, and to look for other signs of injury. This is especially important in the unconcious patient, as ocular injury and retrobulbar haemorrhage may easily be overlooked. *Superficial* foreign bodies such as contact lenses can also be removed. However, if a penetrating injury to the eye is suspected, pressure should be avoided. A dilated pupil may often be due to

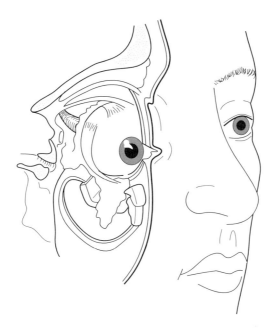

Figure 11.7   Blowout fractures.

local injury, but its significance in relation to head injuries must also be remembered, especially in drowsy patients.

Where there is less swelling, eye movements also need to be documented accurately (orthoptic assessment). CT scans of the orbit enable fractures to be visualized as well as the presence of trapped soft tissues and injuries to the eye itself.

Treatment

Undisplaced fractures of the orbital walls are managed with antibiotics, avoidance of nose blowing, and observation. Indications for surgery include the following:

- retrobulbar haemorrhage (RBH) (see Chapter 10);
- restricted eye movements;
- enophthalmus following a 'blowout fracture';
- large defects on CT or MRI scans.

Surgery aims to decompress the eye (RBH), free trapped tissues and correct the orbital volume by reducing the fractures. If any of the orbital walls are severely damaged they can be repaired using bone, cartilage, lyodermis or synthetic materials. Depending on extent the orbit can be approached via a scalp incision in the hairline (coronal flap) (Fig. 11.8) or a number of direct approaches (e.g. blepharoplasty, trans-conjunctival, or infra-orbital). The timing of surgery varies from unit to unit. Where the fracture is minimal,

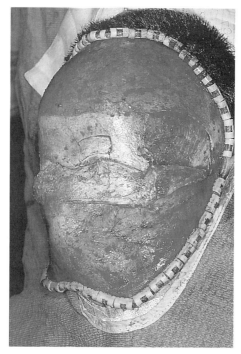

Figure 11.8 Coronal flap. By 'scalping' the patient, this provides excellent exposure of the entire upper facial skeleton, enabling good reduction of bony fragments whilst avoiding incisions on the face.

surgery may be delayed for up to 10–14 days to allow the swelling to settle and CT scans to be ordered. However, if there is obvious evidence of entrapment, surgery may be performed much earlier in order to prevent scarring. Steroids (e.g. dexamethasone) and antibiotics are often given to reduce swelling and prevent life-threatening infection developing from the adjacent sinuses.

Post-operative care is essentially the same as that for zygomatic fractures.

Nasal fractures

These are common, but may be associated with more severe naso-orbitalethmoidal fractures. The nasal skeleton is composed of both bone and cartilage, both of which may be involved. In addition to nasal deformity, the nasal septum may become displaced, resulting in difficulty in breathing through the nose on one side. Epistaxis and a septal haematoma (see Chapter 10) require urgent attention, otherwise treatment can be delayed for up to several weeks in order to allow the swelling to settle. If the patient presents early and with minimal swelling, the nose may be manipulated under anaesthetic on the next available list.

Most fractures are treated by 'closed' reduction, where the bones and, if necessary, the septum are repositioned using forceps. Bleeding from this is common, and often requires nasal packs overnight. The nose is splinted for around 1 to 2 weeks using either plaster of Paris or some other form of mouldable splint. In some cases, if there is an existing laceration over the nose, ORIF using microplates may be carried out. Old fractures may be 'rebroken' and reset in a better position (nasal osteotomy) together with resection of part of the deviated septum (submucous resection, SMR) to allow this to be straightened (see Chapter 15).

General points in management

To maintain the patency of the airway, the patient should be nursed upright. This helps to reduce swelling and discomfort. It should be explained that the surgical repair of the fracture site will necessitate the use of a nasal splint, secured by surgical tape. Intranasal packs may be required for 48–72 h to support the repair, thereby rendering nasal breathing impossible. The patient is less likely to panic when they wake up from the anaesthetic if they are aware of the possibility of nasal packs pre-operatively.

Swelling is usually maximal 48 h post-operatively. Often both eyes and cheeks bruise, and eye care and eye observations may be indicated if the swelling is severe. It is important to ensure that the nasal splint is not rubbing in the inner canthal region, causing a pressure sore. Nasal packs may be left *in situ* for up to 72 h if an immediate septoplasty is performed. A gauze pad can be gently taped under the nostrils to catch any oozing caused by intranasal surgery, and may gently be changed as required.

The nasal packs should be removed with the patient resting quietly on the bed in a semi-recumbent position. The packs should slip out easily, but very gentle tension may be required to remove a stubborn pack. In the event of it proving difficult to remove, medical assistance will be required. It is quite common for the nose to ooze slightly on removal of the packs, so a nasal gauze pad or 'bolster' should be applied under the nostrils and the patient should be encouraged to lie quietly until the bleeding subsides. Patients may quite often feel faint when the packs are removed, so close observation of the patient should be maintained during the recovery period. Once the oozing has stopped, the nares can be very gently cleaned using gauze or a cotton bud but it is vital that neither is pushed into the nostril, as this can cause bleeding to start again, or it may disturb the operation site. The patient should be taught how to care for their nose prior to discharge.

If a plaster of Paris splint is used, and both this and the securing tape have become soiled by oozing, it is possible to discharge the patient home with a relatively clean splint by painting it over with type-correction fluid and leaving it to dry. The original tape should not be removed, as this may disturb the splint, but a fresh piece can be placed over the soiled areas.

The patient must keep their eyes clean in order to ease any discomfort caused by swelling. Regular mouth care using a toothbrush and toothpaste is essential to prevent the delicate oral mucosa from drying out due to mouth breathing. For the 7–10 days that the nasal splint is *in situ*, a soft diet is encouraged to reduce the risk of dislodging the repair. On removal of the splint, the patient may gradually return to a normal diet, but hard chewing should be avoided for up to 6 weeks.

On removal of the splint, the skin across the nose and cheeks is often dry and itchy. The patient can be advised to wash their face as normal and to keep the skin soft and supple by applying a moisturizing cream twice daily. Make-up can be applied when the dryness has disappeared, but a heavy foundation cream, for example, may irritate the skin. Occasionally, the skin may feel numb for a few weeks following the injury and surgery, but sensation usually returns within 3–4 months. Care should be taken when out in the sun to use a high-factor sunblock to reduce the risk of sunburn. Swelling quickly reduces over the 7–10 days, but a residual swelling may remain in the inner canthal region and across the nasal bridge for up to 3 months.

The nose may remain delicate for up to 8 weeks post-operatively, so the patient is advised to avoid contact sports during this time. They should also be advised to avoid sneezing, stooping and smoky environments, all of which can irritate the delicate nasal lining, until a final review is held at 3 months.

Naso-orbitalethmoid and frontal sinus fractures

These injuries effectively involve the bones between the eyes (nasal and ethmoid) and associated structures (frontal sinus, orbits, eyes, canthal ligaments and nasolacrimal apparatus). The fractures are often complex and comminuted, and occur after severe facial and head injuries. They may also extend into the anterior cranial fossa, resulting in CSF leakage.

The medial canthal ligaments may become detached, resulting in an increased distance between the 'corners of the eye' (medial canthi) – telecanthus. These need to be repositioned accurately (canthopexy) if the normal appearances are to be restored. In severe cases the whole orbit may be shifted (orbital dystopia), with gross disfigurement and double vision. The frontal sinuses drain into the nose and, if blocked, this may result in sinusitis and cyst formation. The aims of treatment are therefore:

- to restore facial appearance and function;
- to prevent infection (including meningitis);
- to prevent cyst formation in the frontal sinus.

Treatment

Nasoethmoid-orbital fractures are among the most challenging maxillofacial injuries to treat. In general, the best results are obtained when reconstruction is carried out early. Late correction is extremely difficult. The bones are usually extensively fragmented with significant soft tissue injuries. Surgery is required in the majority of cases, and a number of approaches are available to reduce and fix these fractures. Simple fractures may be managed by nasal splints. However, accurate repositioning of the canthi is essential for a good cosmetic result. Internal fixation is therefore often necessary, either via local incisions or more commonly via a coronal flap (Fig. 11.8). The bones can then be anatomically repositioned and fixed with microplates or titanium mesh.

Fractures of the mid-face

These are significant and varied injuries. Classically, fractures have been described as occurring at three levels, namely Le Fort I, II and III, although often they may be mixed or more extensive. Le Fort II and III fractures involve the orbit, naso-ethmoid region and the base of the skull (Fig. 11.9).

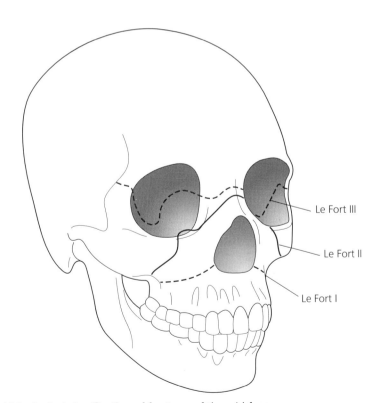

Figure 11.9 Le Fort classification of fractures of the mid-face.

Clinical features include:

- gross swelling with potential airway risk;
- elongation of the face;
- flattening of the profile;
- panda eyes;
- abnormal bite.

Treatment

Most cases require fixation, although in cases where the bones are undisplaced and stable or extensively comminuted and in the frail or in children, they may be treated conservatively (antibiotics, and avoidance of nose-blowing). External fixation was formerly often used for severe injuries. This involved attaching a frame to the skull and using it to support the maxilla until healing had taken place. However, this method has been largely replaced by open reduction and internal fixation using plates, although it may still be appropriate in some cases.

Plates are placed along the 'buttresses' of the mid-face via the mouth, using the bite as a guide to positioning. IMF is usually unnecessary, and early jaw function can be encouraged. Alternatively, suspension wires (circumzygomatic, infra-orbital or frontal) may be used, but may require IMF for 2–4 weeks post-operatively. In Le Fort II fractures skin incisions may be required to reduce the infra-orbital margin and orbital floor. A coronal flap is required for Le Fort II and Le Fort III fractures when the root of the nose and the upper part of the orbits need fixing (Fig. 11.10).

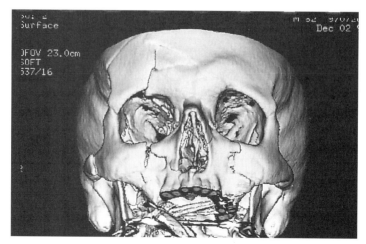

Figure 11.10 Three-dimensional CT scan showing extensive mid-facial fractures extending into the orbits and skull.

General points in management

The patient should be nursed upright to reduce swelling and minimize discomfort, unless other injuries contraindicate this position. Strong analgesia which may depress the level of consciousness or the respiration rate should be avoided. If conscious, patients will usually maintain their airway unaided. However, it should be recognized that they can quickly become exhausted with the effort to keep the airway patent, so close observation is crucial.

Neurological and eye observations are crucial both pre-operatively and post-operatively (see above). The face is usually very swollen and the eyes may be closed due to the severity of the swelling, but manual opening of the eyelids is to be encouraged to monitor visual acuity. Enophthalmus may be present pre-operatively, and a visual acuity chart is required to measure post-operative recovery. Any change in eye observations or neurological status must be reported immediately to the medical staff.

In a Le Fort II or Le Fort III fracture, the cribriform plate fracture usually tears the dura and a cerebrospinal fluid leak can be expected. This tear usually heals spontaneously within 7–10 days, so surgery is rarely required to correct it. Signs of meningitis may become apparent, but it is a rare complication. Mid-face fractures may also fracture into the mouth, sinuses and nasal cavities, and it may be difficult to detect cerebrospinal fluid leakage through rhinorrhoea alone.

The patient will automatically be breathing via their mouth, so oral hygiene is very important to keep them comfortable. Mouth care should be offered and performed hourly to help prevent the delicate oral mucosa from drying out, and to help reduce the risk of infection. The use of toothpaste and toothbrush may not be possible pre-operatively, so mouthwashes must be used. The lips should be kept moist with petroleum jelly to prevent them from cracking and becoming sore.

Pre-operatively, patients may be unable or unwilling to eat. An intravenous infusion is usually started and a fluid-balance chart commenced. Drinking is possible in some cases, but most patients are reluctant to try. If the patient is able to drink, this will help to keep their mouth moist and comfortable.

Post-operatively, dietary requirements are important, and a visit from the dietitian is helpful in working out an individual nutritional assessment plan. A high-calorie, high-protein diet is to be encouraged. Most patients can manage a soft or liquid diet. Mid-face fractures are usually plated or wired internally, so care is needed when eating not to put too much pressure on the repair site. The patient should be advised about weight loss during the recovery period of 4–6 weeks, but as a normal diet is again tolerated, so the lost weight will be regained.

Facial sutures are removed between 3 and 7 days, depending on the site. Scalp staples (following coronal incision) can be removed at 7 to 10 days. Patients may complain of numbness in the face once the swelling has subsided but, over a period of months, sensation will return to a greater or lesser degree.

Psychological support for the patient and their family is important. It should be explained that the vascularity in the face results in so much swelling and bruising but that it all settles quickly, often within 7–10 days. However, the appearance can be very upsetting for all concerned, although post-operatively the face should be restored to a good pre-injury likeness. Post-traumatic symptoms may include nightmares as a result of the injury. These usually diminish with time, but support may be required for a while, and family, friends and carers should be aware of this.

The patient should be encouraged to avoid smoky environments, stooping, sneezing or any other activity that could irritate the delicate mucosa. Contact sports and heavy lifting should also be discouraged until the repairs have had time to start to mature, usually at 6–10 weeks.

Dento-alveolar injuries

This includes injuries to the teeth and their supporting bone.

Injuries to the teeth themselves range from chips off the enamel to crown or root fractures involving the tooth pulp. The periodontal ligament and surrounding 'gum' support the teeth in their sockets and cushion the chewing forces. These may be 'concussed' (injury without loosening). Alternatively, intact teeth may be intruded (driven into the bone), displaced or avulsed (pulled out of the socket). Fractures of the supporting alveolar bone may or may not be associated.

Treatment is required when there is:

- pain or sensitivity to hot and cold;
- recent avulsion or displacement;
- mobility;
- alveolar bone fracture;
- cosmetic deformity.

The principles of treatment include:

- pain relief;
- control of bleeding;
- dressing of exposed dentine or pulp;
- repositioning/replantation of the tooth, which is then splinted for a variable time depending on the nature of the injury;
- reduction and fixation of alveolar bone;
- cosmetic repair.

Where there is minimal displacement and mobility and the patient can bite normally these can be managed in a similar way to mandibular fractures. In more extensive fractures treatment may require:

- removal of the fragments;
- fixation using arch bars or plastic splints;
- open reduction and fixation with plates or wires.

If the teeth on the fragment are damaged they will require appropriate attention. If they need to be removed this is sometimes delayed until the fracture has healed, in order to keep the blood supply to the segment. Treatment is often prolonged, and usually requires endodontic treatment (root filling) at a later stage.

12 Head and neck malignancy

Michael Perry and Caroline Evans

This chapter will describe those tumours of the head and neck that are commonly seen in maxillofacial practice. These include those arising in:

- the mouth – oral cancer;
- skin;
- bone;
- salivary tissue (see Chapter 13).

Oral cancer

'Oral cancer' refers to a group of tumours involving the lips, oral cavity and oropharynx (Fig. 12.1). This includes:

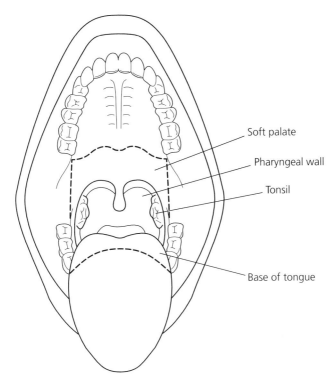

Soft palate

Pharyngeal wall

Tonsil

Base of tongue

Figure 12.1 The oral cavity and oropharynx.

- squamous-cell carcinoma (SCC);
- tumours arising from minor salivary glands;
- lymphomas;
- malignant melanomas;
- sarcomas;
- primary intra-osseous carcinoma;
- metastases.

Over 85 per cent of oral cancers are squamous-cell carcinoma (SCC). Tumours arising from the salivary glands in the lips and mouth (not including the major salivary glands; see Chapter 13) represent the second largest group.

SCC is the commonest cancer of the upper aerodigestive tract (the internal nose, mouth, pharynx, oesophagus and trachea). World-wide it is the sixth commonest cancer, accounting for up to 40 per cent of all tumours in the Indian subcontinent. However, in the UK it only accounts for 1–2 per cent of all tumours. Around 3.5 new patients in every 100 000 are seen each year, placing it in about 15th position on a 'league table' of cancer sites in males, and in about 20th position for females. This is equivalent to around 2000 new cases registered each year. Overall, only about 50 per cent of patients with oral cancer are still alive after 5 years. The total number of deaths each year is therefore similar to that for those who die from breast cancer, cervical cancer and malignant melanoma.

Oral cancer appears to be increasing in young patients and in females. In addition, a significant number of patients (in some reports up to 20 per cent) go on to develop a *second* carcinoma in the upper aerodigestive tract. If current trends continue at the present rate, oral cancer will become a significant health problem. Such an increase may be partly due to the large rise in alcohol consumption in the UK.

When it is diagnosed and treated early, oral cancer is a curable disease. However, many patients still present with advanced disease due to delays in diagnosis. Treatment of advanced lesions is associated with significant physical and psychological complications, whereas small lesions are relatively simple to deal with. Carcinoma of the posterior one-third of the tongue in particular has a poor prognosis, because lack of early symptoms and signs leads to late diagnosis.

Treatment of advanced oral cancer often carries a high psychological morbidity. Studies have shown severe effects such as:

- loss of identity;
- grief reaction;
- change in body image and self-image;
- loss of self-esteem and self-confidence;
- feelings of humiliation;
- fear of reactions of other people;
- social withdrawal and isolation;
- family stresses;
- loss of sexuality;
- reactive depression;
- a high proportion do not return to work, or have to change their occupation.

In addition to the alteration of facial appearance, patients also experience problems with salivary control, taste, swallowing, speech, nutrition and mastication.

Death from oral cancer

People die from oral cancer usually as a result of recurrence either at the original 'primary' site or in the neck. However, as control of the disease at these sites improves, death from other metastases (e.g. lung, liver) is becoming more common.

Aetiology

Established risk factors for carcinoma of the oral cavity include the following:

- smoking;
- alcohol;

- betel habits;
- previous aerodigestive malignancy.

Other factors which have been implicated include:

- chronic candidal infection;
- some viral infections;
- oral syphilis;
- alcohol in mouthwashes;
- nutritional and vitamin deficiencies (diets that have an adequate iron, vitamin C and vitamin A analog content are believed to be protective);
- some viruses;
- immunosuppression;
- occupation;
- ethnic origin.

Tobacco, whether smoked or chewed, is the most important risk factor. It may be taken as part of the betel quid in combination with areka nut and lime, although in the UK smoking is by far the commonest form. If smoking is stopped the risk falls over about 15 to 20 years to that for individuals who have never smoked. Alcohol is also a significant risk factor for oral and pharyngeal tumours. Alcohol is often associated with smoking, and heavy drinkers who also smoke carry a very high risk. These effects appear to be multiplicative, not additive.

Epstein–Barr virus (EBV) infection is associated with Burkitt's lymphoma, a malignant tumour which can affect the jaws. EBV is also associated with nasopharyngeal carcinoma. Other viruses (e.g. human papilloma virus (HPV) and herpes simplex virus (HSV)), may have a role, but this has not yet been proven. Patients who are immunosuppressed due to AIDS may present with Kaposi's sarcoma.

Some studies suggest that nutritional factors may be important in the development of oropharyngeal cancer. Low intake of vitamins A and C is associated with an increased risk. Diets with a high content of raw yellow or green vegetables and fresh fruits are said to be protective, and supplementation with various vitamins is claimed to be protective. The most consistent dietary findings are the protective effects of high levels of fruit consumption and the risks of high alcohol intake. Cultural dietary practices (e.g. wood-stove cooking and a high intake of chilli powder) are claimed to be important. Dietary iron may also play a role in maintaining healthy mucosa and thus reducing susceptibility to cancer. High fat consumption is also claimed to be a strong risk factor for oral cancer.

Exposure to wood dust, organic chemicals, coal products and cement have all been suggested as risk factors for some oropharyngeal and laryngeal cancers.

Some oral conditions are described as 'potentially malignant or premalignant', in that they occasionally predispose to oral cancer. These include the following:

- leukoplakia;
- erythroplakia;
- speckled leukoplakia (mixture of the above);
- erosive lichen planus;
- oral submucous fibrosis;
- chronic sideropenia.

About 25 per cent of cancers are preceded by these 'potentially malignant lesions', especially erythroplakia, leukoplakia and speckled leukoplakia. It has been estimated that oral leukoplakia and erythroplasia carry a 3 to 6 per cent risk of malignant transformation.

Clinical features and spread of disease

Oral cancer can occur anywhere in the mouth, but is most commonly seen (in descending order of frequency) in the following areas (see Fig. 12.1):

- the anterior two-thirds of the tongue;
- the floor of the mouth;
- just behind the wisdom teeth (retromolar trigone);
- on the cheek;
- on the palate.

Carcinoma of the lip will be considered with skin cancers later. The floor of the mouth and the under-surface of the tongue are by far the commonest sites that act as a reservoir for carcinogens, allowing prolonged exposure.

Most patients present with a single 'primary' tumour. However, some present with *multiple* primary malignancies in the aerodigestive tract (e.g. carcinoma of the tongue with carcinoma of the lung), known as 'simultaneous' cancers. If the second tumour occurs within 6 months of the first it is described as a 'synchronous' cancer, whereas if it occurs after 6 months it is said to be 'metachronous'. Other patients present with involvement of the cervical lymph nodes in the neck from an 'occult' cancer in the orofacial region.

The symptoms and signs of oral cancer are highly variable (see Box 12.1) (Figs 12.2 and 12.3). However, pain is unusual, although it may be present in advanced cancers which have spread into neighbouring tissues, affecting swallowing and speech. Small tumours cause few symptoms and therefore patients often present with advanced disease. For these reasons, *all unexplained non-healing ulcers and 'rashes' should undergo biopsy after only a short period of observation (2 to 3 weeks)*. Of course many of these symptoms may be due to other benign conditions such as periodontal disease, *so a high index of suspicion is essential.*

Tumours initially spread locally, and distant spread is a late feature. Those that arise on the gingiva (gums) may spread into the jaw via the tooth sockets, invading bone and loosening the teeth.

The spread of cancer to the lymph nodes in the neck is often predictable, depending partly on where the primary tumour arises (Fig. 12.4). The

BOX 12.1   Symptoms and signs of oral cancer

- Pain
- Ulceration
- Swelling
- Lump
- Contact bleeding
- Loose teeth
- Numbness of the lip or tongue
- Difficulty with speech and swallowing
- Loss of weight
- Incidental finding (e.g. potentially malignant lesion, painless ulcer)
- Trismus
- Bad breath

likelihood of involvement depends on tumour size, site and aggressiveness. Generally speaking, larger and more aggressive tumours that are further back in the mouth are more likely to have spread to the lymph nodes when seen. Cervical nodes are grouped into five levels (Fig. 12.5), through which spread occurs in a stepwise fashion. 'Level one' is usually involved first, before the lower levels. If the upper levels are normal, the likelihood of the others being involved is very low. Most studies show that involvement of the cervical nodes by tumour is one of the major factors determining survival.

Assessment

A full history, including a history of risk factors, is essential. Not only are smoking habits and alcohol consumption important for assessing the risk of oral

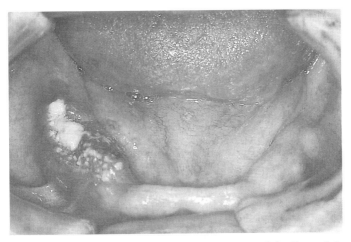

Figure 12.2   Oropharyngeal cancer. Squamous-cell carcinoma of the floor of the mouth.

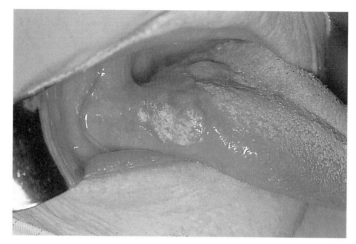

Figure 12.3 Oropharyngeal cancer. Squamous-cell carcinoma of the lateral border of the tongue.

cancer, but they are also associated with risks of general anaesthesia (see Chapter 1). Thorough examination of the mouth, throat, dental status and neck is also necessary, which may include an examination under general anaesthesia. Good lighting is required, particularly when examining the 'coffin corner' (posterior tongue/floor of mouth). This is a site where small tumours can easily be missed.

Examination of the neck is a well-recognized problem, particularly in the case of necks which are fat or thick-set. Further investigations such as computed tomography (CT) (Fig. 12.6), magnetic resonance imaging (MRI) and ultrasound-guided fine-needle aspiration may be necessary. The size of the primary tumour can also be assessed with CT or MRI. Plain radiographs are

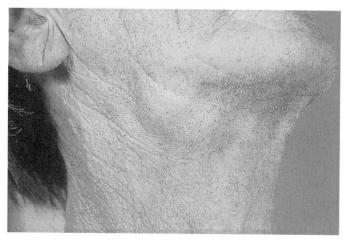

Figure 12.4 Submandibular swelling. This patient presented with swelling in the region of the submandibular gland. This was the presenting feature of an oral cancer.

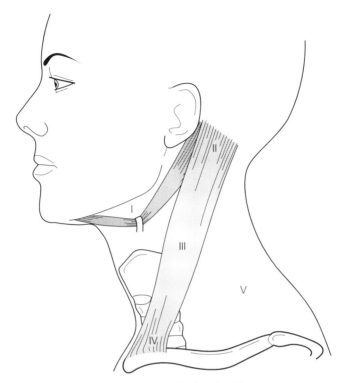

Figure 12.5 Subdivision of cervical lymph nodes (levels I–V).

useful for assessing the teeth. Very detailed screening of patients for distant metastases is usually unnecessary, although a chest X-ray and liver function tests may be required.

Incisional biopsy (see Chapter 8) is mandatory prior to treatment planning.

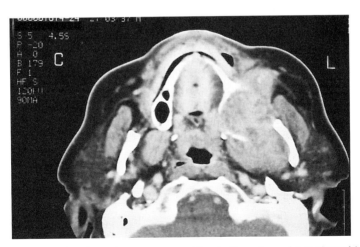

Figure 12.6 CT scan showing a large tumour arising in the retromolar region which has penetrated and destroyed adjacent bone.

Lymphomas, for example, are best treated with radiotherapy even when advanced. Examination under general anaesthesia is usually required in advanced disease to assess the size of the tumour and the involvement of deeper structures. This also entails oesophagoscopy, gastroscopy, laryngoscopy and bronchoscopy, during which the whole of the upper aerodigestive tract is visualized in order to look for simultaneous tumours. At the same time, where there has been much weight loss or where feeding in the post-operative period is expected to be difficult, this provides an opportunity to carry out a percutaneous gastrostomy (PEG) to provide nutritional support. Other procedures, such as extractions of diseased teeth, may also be carried out, particularly where radiotherapy seems likely.

Management

The management of oral cancer requires a multidisciplinary team. It is important to consider not only the disease but also the patient's general physical, psychological and social status. Not only do patients have to face the fear of dying, but also they have fears of disfigurement and of loss of speech and swallowing following treatment. The team should therefore include a surgeon, radiotherapist, trained nurse/counsellors (e.g. Macmillan and Marie Curie nurses), dietitians, speech therapists, physiotherapists, maxillofacial technicians, dental hygienists and restorative/prosthetic specialists. General medical and dental practitioners and also medical social workers should be involved as well. Home-help and other support services are often required.

Most patients are now treated in 'cancer units' or 'cancer centres' in the UK, an approach which enables co-ordination of treatment, rehabilitation and psychological and social support. As recommended in the 'policy framework for commissioning cancer services', any surgeons involved should be specialists in the anatomical area in question.

The two main treatment options are radiotherapy and surgery. These are often used in combination, although preferences for each vary between treatment centres. They should be regarded as complementary treatments rather than competing ones. Whichever option is used for the initial treatment, the alternative may be reserved for 'salvage' should recurrence occur later.

Prior to treatment, patients are usually seen in 'oncology' clinics where all members of the team are available. This enables a joint decision to be made on the best treatment and any pre-operative/pre-radiotherapy procedures to be planned (e.g. extractions, PEG insertion, etc.). At the same time, if necessary further investigations can be ordered as part of the 'work-up' for theatre.

Generally speaking, with advanced disease or where there is evidence of bone invasion and/or spread to the cervical lymph node, surgery is considered to be appropriate, followed by post-operative radiotherapy. Bone reduces the effectiveness of radiotherapy, and its involvement is therefore usually an indication for surgery. For small, well-localized soft tissue tumours either surgery or radiotherapy can be used although surgery is preferred if deformity or functional problems are unlikely, as it is quicker. Intermediate-sized tumours benefit equally from either treatment, and it is here that opinions vary most.

Surgery

The aims of surgery are:

- to remove completely the tumour and any involved cervical nodes;
- to reconstruct missing tissues, enabling functional rehabilitation;
- minimal complications.

Admission

Since most patients are middle-aged or older, often with a long history of smoking or alcohol consumption, there is usually some anaesthetic risk. They therefore need to be thoroughly assessed prior to surgery, and are sometimes admitted 1–2 days beforehand to enable investigations to be carried out (see Chapter 1). This also gives the anaesthetist an opportunity to see the patient in good time and to advise on further treatment (pre-operative physiotherapy, nebulizers, antibiotics, etc.). The following must be considered:

- nebulizers;
- antibiotics (on induction);
- DVT prophylaxis (e.g. heparin, TED stockings);
- stress ulcer prophylaxis (e.g. ranitidine);
- steroids to reduce swelling;
- pain control/anti-emetics;
- prophylaxis for alcohol withdrawal;
- assessment by dietitian and speech and language specialist;
- general morale.

Tumour resection

Particular care of the airway is important in all patients undergoing major surgery, particularly those with bilateral neck dissection, which may require a tracheostomy.

Some small tumours (e.g. on the side of the tongue, palate or cheek) may be simply excised and the resulting raw area left to heal. Alternatively, these tumours may be treated with radiotherapy. With palatal tumours, 'dressing plates' can be made to cover the palate, which can then be lined with a sedative dressing such as Coe-pack. These wounds heal surprisingly quickly, and dressing plates are often only needed for a few weeks.

Larger tumours require some kind of reconstruction to facilitate rehabilitation (see below). Improvements in surgical access now mean that previously 'irresectable' tumours (e.g. posterior tongue) are no longer considered to be so. These can now be completely excised under direct vision. For example, tumours in the back of the mouth, soft palate and pharynx can be accessed via a 'mandibulotomy' (Figs 12.7 and 12.8). Here the lower lip is split and the mandible 'osteotomized' or divided between the teeth, allowing the two halves to be separated rather like the pages of a book. Osteotomy of the maxilla through an upper lip incision extending up alongside the nose aids access to the posterior part of the palate and retromaxillary region. Following tumour excision these bones can be repositioned and fixed using miniplates. Careful placement of the incisions and good post-operative wound care now leave virtually invisible scars in the majority of patients.

BOX 12.2 Surgical access for 'deep' head and neck tumours

Many approaches are described. These include the following:
1 Transfacial
   • Pedicled osteotomy of the maxilla, hard palate and zygoma
   • Maxillary osteotomy
   • Nasal osteotomy
2 Le Fort I osteotomy
3 Lip split/mandibular split
4 Lateral zygomatic osteotomy
5 Lateral orbitotomy
6 Via the cranial base (see below)

Greater understanding of bone invasion means that it is now possible, in selected cases, to preserve the lower border of the mandible, thereby maintaining facial contour. Where there is no evidence of bone invasion, extensive jaw resection is not necessary. Instead, where the tumour sits on the mandible

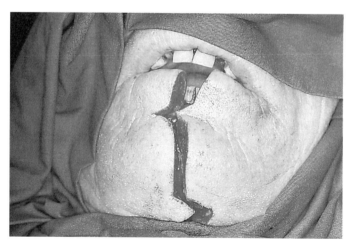

Figure 12.7 Mandibulotomy. Lip split prior to division of mandible.

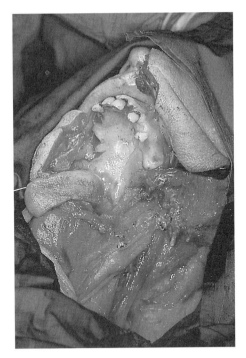

Figure 12.8 Mandibulotomy. This provides excellent exposure of the base of the tongue, the pharynx and the soft palate.

but does not appear to involve it, a 'marginal resection' where the lower border is left may be carried out. Because sufficient healthy bone must remain to avoid fracture, this technique is difficult to apply to the edentulous, thin mandible. Where bone is clearly involved, segmental 'block resection' of the jaw is necessary. Here the full thickness of the mandible is excised in the region of the tumour, resulting in a permanently numb lower lip. In most cases the ramus and temporomandibular joint (TMJ) are preserved, the latter being particularly important for good jaw function.

Neck dissection

This refers to the removal of lymph nodes in the neck which 'drain' the head and neck area. Microscopic tumour cells can pass to these nodes, where they become lodged and grow as 'regional' metastases.

For many years 'radical' neck dissection was the only operation considered to be effective in removing these nodes (Fig. 12.9). This involves resecting the lymph nodes together with the sternomastoid muscle, internal jugular vein, accessory nerve and submandibular gland. However, this is accompanied by problems due to loss of the accessory nerve resulting in a painful stiff shoulder. Where both sides of the neck are dissected, gross and long-lasting swelling of the head occurs, severely compromising the airway and necessitating the placement of a tracheostomy. Over the years, modifications in the

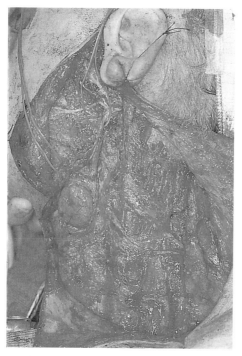

Figure 12.9 Radical neck dissection.

extent of surgery have become possible due to better understanding of the patterns of spread. Preservation of these structures may now be undertaken, thereby reducing post-operative complications. The terminology has accordingly become quite complex!

Where the cervical nodes are thought to be involved (by examination or on CT), a neck dissection is usually required which may be either 'radical' (with wide clearance) or 'functional' (preservation of key structures), depending on the extent of involvement. However, the management of *clinically normal* necks is more controversial, since surgery is not without risk. In these cases, approximately one-third of patients with small tumours will in fact have microscopic deposits in the nodes, usually in the upper three levels. The likelihood of metastases depends on several factors, such as the site of the primary tumour, its size and the depth of invasion. Determination of the overall risk of spread is therefore essential, as involvement of the cervical nodes is the most important prognostic factor in head and neck cancer. If they are involved, survival is reduced by 50 per cent when compared to similar tumours without metastases.

Many surgeons now prefer preventive treatment of clinically and CT/MRI normal necks, either surgically or by radiotherapy. In these patients a 'supraomohyoid' neck dissection is undertaken in which the upper three levels are removed. This enables microscopic examination of the nodes, which helps to determine the need for post-operative radiotherapy.

Reconstruction

A bewildering number of reconstructive techniques is available, the final choice depending on the size and site of the defect, bone involvement, the general health of the patient (e.g. can they withstand a long anaesthetic?) and whether there has been previous radiotherapy to the area. Tissue can be taken from local sites (e.g. nasolabial flaps, temporalis flaps) or distant sites (e.g. 'free flaps' or pectoralis muscle flaps).

BOX 12.3   Some examples of 'flaps' that are commonly used in head and neck reconstruction

- Nasolabial
- Temporalis
- Glabellar flap
- Buccal fat pad
- Delto pectoral
- Pectoralis major
- Latissimus dorsi
- 'Free flaps'

BOX 12.4   Properties of different flaps

'Pedicled' flaps (e.g. nasolabial, pectoralis major). These are flaps which have a well-defined 'axial' blood supply on which survival of the flap initially depends. They are therefore raised on a small pedicle through which these vessels pass. So long as the axial vessels are not kinked or damaged as the flap is raised and repositioned, large amounts of skin can be used.

'Random pattern' flaps. These rely on numerous and unpredictable small vessels to keep the tissues alive. They therefore require a broad attachment at the base if necrosis of the distal end is to be avoided. Since the skin of the head and neck has an excellent blood supply, the success rate of local flaps is generally very high.

'Free tissue transfer' ('free' flaps, see below). Tissues from remote parts of the body (e.g. skin, muscle, bone, and occasionally bowel or omentum) can be used in head and neck reconstruction. The tissues are raised together with their feeding blood vessels (pedicle), which are separated from the donor site. The 'free' flap can then be used for reconstruction, the blood vessels being 'plumbed in' (anastamosed) to suitable vessels in the neck. This technique has greatly increased the variety of tissues available for reconstruction, with improved functional and cosmetic results.

When the mandible is involved, the objective is to restore function and cosmesis completely. Psychological studies have shown an inverse relationship between the ability to chew properly and both body image satisfaction and depression. It is also essential to provide a functioning prosthesis as early as possible after surgery. The major problem following total or subtotal glossectomy is related to loss of the tongue muscles that are necessary for swallowing and speech. Tongue volume can be replaced using bulky flaps (e.g. rectus abdominus or latissimus dorsi), but significant movement is unlikely. Surgery of the palate can lead to speech difficulties and prevention of regurgitation into the nose during swallowing. In general, the use of an obturator (with or without a speech appliance) or reconstructive surgery is required, but these often fail to restore the patient's speech completely. Full-thickness cheek reconstruction involving the corner of the mouth is particularly difficult, and it is essential to maintain the sphincter-like function that is essential for eating.

Tumour resection should never be compromised by the reconstructive technique. Complete removal is the first consideration. The use of 'free tissue transfer' using microvascular anastomosis now means that virtually all defects can be reconstructed. With safe anaesthesia it is now possible to carry out reconstruction of the mandible, maxilla and mucosa at the same time as the resection. For larger defects, free vascularized tissues provide the best chance for functional rehabilitation. By using healthy vascularized tissue, wound healing is improved and, where necessary, implant-retained dentures can aid oral rehabilitation (see Chapter 16). Pedicled flaps (e.g. pectoralis major) are useful but bulky, and restrict tongue movement. Bone grafts (e.g. ribs) and large titanium 'reconstruction' plates have a limited role in the mandibular reconstruction in the frail patient, but ideally should be avoided in cases where radiotherapy is likely to be required afterwards.

Many free flaps have been described. Those commonly used in the oral cavity include:

- composite radial forearm flaps (Figs 12.10 and 12.11);
- deep circumflex iliac artery flaps (vascularized hip grafts);
- fibula flaps;
- scapula flaps.

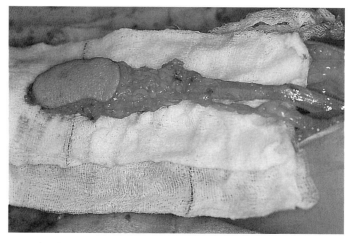

Figure 12.10   Radial forearm fasciocutaneous free flap still attached to the forearm by the radial artery and cephalic vein.

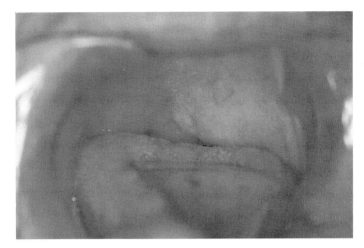

Figure 12.11 Radial forearm free flap used to reconstruct soft palate following excision of tumour.

Each flap consists of a variable amount of skin and bone to enable reconstruction of bone and mucosa. Each flap has its own merits and complications associated with the donor site. Bone quality also varies, and this needs to be taken into account when considering the use of osseointegrated implants (see Chapter 16).

The composite radial forearm free flap is commonly used, and is capable of providing skin and a strut of bone up to around 15 cm long. Post-operatively the patient needs to wear a plaster cast as the radius can fracture if it is not protected. Bone from the pelvis (deep circumflex iliac flap) has also become popular. The thick bone provides good support for implants, and it can also be used in reconstruction of the maxilla.

The survival of free flaps depends on a good blood supply through the feeding vessels, which are usually anastamosed to vessels in the neck. Thrombosis at the anastamosis is very uncommon, but when it does occur requires urgent revision if the flap is to be saved. Frequent (initially hourly) post-operative monitoring is therefore essential in the early post-operative period. Most flaps fail within the first 5 days, although there are occasional exceptions. Most units rely on clinical assessment, although this is very observer-dependent. Research continues into more objective methods of assessment, and many non-invasive methods have been devised. These essentially involve monitoring the partial pressure of oxygen, blood flow through the flap, temperature, tissue pH or energy metabolism. Doppler ultrasound, intracutaneous pO_2 measurement and spectrophotometry have all been suggested (see Chapter 9).

Rehabilitation following maxillary resections

Rehabilitation after resection of the maxilla (e.g. for SCC of the alveolus or antrum) can be achieved by the use of either an obturator, a local flap (e.g.

temporalis flap) or a vascularized flap (e.g. deep circumflex iliac artery). The choice varies from unit to unit.

The advantages of flaps include the following:

- immediate reconstruction with minimal post-operative supervision;
- avoidance of the discomfort and nasal reflux which may occur with a poorly fitting obturator;
- it is psychologically better for the patient.

The disadvantages include the following:

- a defect in the donor area;
- construction of a denture to fit over the flap may be difficult;
- early detection of tumour recurrence is difficult;
- some patients develop catarrh or nasal stuffiness.

The advantages of obturators are as follows:

- removal allows early detection of tumour recurrence;
- good cheek support;
- well-designed obturator fits better than dentures constructed over a large flap.

The disadvantages are as follows:

- obturators can be quite bulky and may be difficult to insert;
- frequent adjustment is necessary;
- crusting of the surgical defect may distress the patient and require frequent removal;
- patients may find it distasteful to remove a large prosthesis, and they may also find that the residual defect is a constant reminder of the cancer.

BOX 12.5 Complications of surgery

- Bleeding
- General infections (e.g. chest, urine, etc.)
- Local infections (wound, plates)
- Wound breakdown, sinus or fistula formation, which may require further surgery and can delay radiotherapy
- Post-operative leakage of chyle into the neck wound
- Prolonged post-operative pain
- Flap necrosis
- DVT
- Incomplete excision
- Excessive scarring of facial skin or soft tissue deformity
- Failure to restore the occlusion
- Complications at donor sites

Salvage surgery

This is surgery required for recurrent disease following unsuccessful radio-therapy and/or previous surgery. Recurrence is usually at the site of the primary tumour or in the cervical nodes. However, advances in imaging techniques, enabling earlier detection, and improved surgical techniques now mean that successful salvage surgery has become possible in more cases.

Cranial base surgery

Tumours may spread to involve the skull base (anterior and middle cranial fossae) or arise from the sinuses (ethmoid, sphenoid and frontal), orbits or infratemporal fossa. In addition, tumours arising from within the skull may spread to involve the skull base. Access to the cranial base therefore requires close teamwork with neurosurgeons and ophthalmologists.

The skull base may be approached in several ways, either from above by means of a frontal craniotomy, or via the face – transfacially, e.g. the Autemere (lateral rotation) or Panje (frontonasal) osteotomies. These approaches are particularly useful for tumours involving the paranasal sinuses and the retromaxillary area. As described in the above section on tumour resection, after skin incisions and bone cuts the maxilla can be rotated outwards like the pages of a book. The use of natural skin creases to place incisions helps to improve the final cosmetic result.

Additional complications of this major surgery include cerebrospinal fluid (CSF) leakage, meningitis and brain injury. Following resection, local or distant flaps are used to seal off the cranial cavity from the sinuses and oral and nasal cavities. This is essential to prevent infection.

Radiotherapy in head and neck cancer

Radiotherapy has an important role in the treatment of early tumours. It is also often used following surgery in the management of advanced cancers. This depends on the histological examination of the resected tissue which defines the adequacy of clearance. When post-operative radiotherapy is required, treatment should ideally start within 4 to 8 weeks of surgery.

Radiotherapy uses ionizing radiation to kill tumour cells by damaging DNA, which is either repaired by the cell or results in mutation or death. Unfortunately, ionizing radiation does not distinguish between normal cells and cancer cells, and both are equally radiosensitive. To kill a tumour with a single dose of radiation, so much would be required that this would result in irreparable damage to the normal tissues. This problem is overcome by treating with smaller daily doses or 'fractions'. Normal cells recover from radiotherapy quicker than cancer cells. By fractionating the doses, cumulative damage occurs in the tumour cells, whilst allowing an adequate time for the normal tissues to recover.

Radiation is obtained either from naturally occurring radioactive isotopes, or from artificially produced X-rays. Some head and neck tumours (e.g. lymphomas) appear to be particularly sensitive to irradiation and surgery is not necessary. Radiotherapy may also be used to reduce symptoms (e.g. to reduce bone pain from metastases).

Side-effects of radiotherapy to the head and neck

With modern equipment and careful planning of the beam direction, most of the former severe side-effects of radiotherapy no longer occur.

BOX 12.6 Side-effects of radiotherapy to the head and neck

- Dermatitis
- Skin erythema with scaling – patients should keep the treated area dry and clean, and avoid using soap
- Stomatitis
- Xerostomia (dry mouth)
- Alopecia (usually temporary)
- Lethargy
- Depression
- Loss of appetite
- Nausea and vomiting
- Osteoradionecrosis
- Radiation-induced cancers, although these are seen 20 years or more after radical therapy and the risk appears to be extremely small

Skin is irradiated in all patients treated with external irradiation. However, using modern techniques most of the dose is delivered at depth and spares the skin. Hair follicles, sweat glands, sebaceous glands and salivary glands may all be damaged.

Late reactions may take months or years to develop. In young patients this may include central nervous system (CNS) demyelination, cataracts and dryness of the eye (following treatment for orbital tumours), requiring the application of artificial tears. Fibrosis of the soft tissues can result in reduced jaw and tongue mobility. Irradiation of the inner ear (e.g. during treatment for nasopharyngeal carcinoma), may damage the cochlea, resulting in hearing loss. Permanent hair loss can occur with high doses targeted directly at skin tumours.

Following irradiation of the oral cavity, patients are frequently predisposed to colonization of the mucosa by yeasts, usually candida. In cases where the salivary glands have been irradiated the risk of candidosis is even higher. A reduction in salivary flow reduces the normal cleansing action of saliva, as well as the amount of mucosal secretory antibodies (IgA). This results in a more favourable environment for candidal adhesion. The incidence of candida in the normal population has been reported to be up to 68 per cent. Following radiotherapy, candida can persist for up to 6 months. Treatment includes the use of topical and occasionally systemic antifungal agents such as Miconozole, Nystatin, Amphetericin B and Fluconazole. Dentures, smoking and alcohol abuse also increase candida colonization. Fungi colonize the dentures, resulting in persistence despite antifungal therapy. Excellent oral hygiene is therefore essential. Dentures should be left out at night to provide 'breathing space' for the mucosa. Antiseptic mouthwashes and the avoidance of smoking and spicy foods are advised. Aspirin mouthwash may be useful in stomatitis, and saliva substitutes are helpful in dysphagia.

Irradiation of the oral cavity can also cause necrosis of bone which can later become infected. This condition is known as osteoradionecrosis (ORN). Once established, this is extremely difficult to manage. ORN is essentially a problem of wound healing rather than infection. Radiation results in hypoxic, hypovascular and hypocellular tissue which breaks down, leaving chronic non-healing wounds. Contamination by bacteria leads to the chronic sepsis of the dead bone. The incidence of osteoradionecrosis has been reported to be up to 37 per cent. The risk increases if teeth (particularly from the mandible) are extracted following treatment. If teeth need to be removed, prophylactic antibiotics and care of the tissues will reduce the risk of infection. All patients with oropharyngeal cancer should therefore have a dental assessment *prior* to treatment. All diseased teeth should then be extracted in good time and oral hygiene improved.

Management of ORN involves the removal of any plates or wires, immobilization of the mandible and surgical debridement. Orocutaneous fistulae will only close once necrotic infected tissues have been removed. To reduce contamination, a nasogastric tube or PEG may be necessary. Fistulae may need to be excised or closed using pedicled or free tissue. Other measures include hyperbaric oxygen, and ultrasound therapy has been suggested. Long-term antibiotics are required. Osteoradionecrosis is now seen less often due to better techniques of administering radiotherapy, which have led to reduced bone absorption.

Chemotherapy

Chemotherapy has no established role in the management of squamous-cell carcinoma, although trials do exist that are evaluating its potential in locally advanced or recurrent disease. Both chemotherapy and fast-neutron therapy have significant side-effects, and to date do not show any increase in survival compared to surgery or radiotherapy. Their use at present should be limited to randomized controlled trials.

Follow-up

Following discharge, early post-operative care requires the support of the general practitioner, practice nurses, social services and specialist services (e.g. the Macmillan nurses and the 'Lets Face It' organization). These arrangements need to be made before the patient is discharged home. All patients should be examined, usually every month for about 1 year after treatment, and then at less frequent intervals in subsequent years.

Any suspicion of a recurrence at the primary site or in the neck, or of a second primary or a distant metastasis needs urgent investigation. Such recurrences usually indicate a poor prognosis for the patient. In the majority of these patients curative treatment is not possible. Palliative care may include further surgery to prevent tumour tissue from fungating and becoming infected. Particular attention needs to be given to the control of symptoms. Adequate analgesia and anti-emetic treatment and wound care are often needed. Specialist care such as the Macmillan nurses and hospice care may be necessary and should be available if needed.

Prevention

Oral cancer is largely a preventable disease in the majority of cases. Patient education regarding tobacco and alcohol-related habits and regular screening by dentists and doctors are essential for reducing the incidence of the disease and enabling its early detection. High-risk groups need to be identified and the opportunity taken to assess cancerous and pre-cancerous changes. Treatment at an early stage is curative and also has fewer complications. Doctors and dentists should avoid unnecessary delays by referring earlier and not treating suspicious lesions with antibiotics, antifungals and mouthwashes. The evidence also suggests that a diet high in trace elements and anti-oxidant vitamins (vitamins A, C and E) is also protective. Enough is known, therefore, to improve society's effectiveness in primary prevention by health promotion and education.

The future

Photodynamic therapy

Photodynamic therapy is a promising treatment currently under investigation as an alternative to surgery and radiotherapy. The process involves the selective destruction of tumours using a photosensitizing agent (dihaematoporphyrine ether) administered systemically, and an argon laser. This releases highly reactive oxygen radicals, causing cell death and tumour necrosis. Tumour cells are relatively more photosensitive, and therefore this process causes less damage to normal tissues. This stage is then followed by tissue regeneration. However, patients need to avoid direct sunlight for 30 days after treatment, as the skin remains photosensitized and exposure to sunlight can cause a severe reaction.

Retinoids

These may be of use in the treatment of oral leukoplakia and in the prevention of cancer. In a number of non-randomized controlled trials using vitamin A and beta-carotene, clinical remission of oral leukoplakia in up to 90 per cent of subjects has been reported.

Immunomodulation

The role of the immune system in the pathogenesis and treatment of cancer is still being investigated. It may be possible that biological response modifiers (BRM) will have therapeutic potential in head and neck cancer, and clinical trials are in progress. Preliminary studies with pre-treated patients have demonstrated antitumour activity, with the suggestion that immunotherapy may provide a treatment alternative.

Molecular genetics

Recent studies have suggested that molecular genetics may help to identify potentially malignant oral lesions. The clinical appearance of these lesions is a poor predictor of progression to invasive cancer. Experimental work on onco-gene activation and tumour suppressor gene inactivation has provided encouraging results by yielding prognostic information.

Exfoliative cytology

Exfoliative cytology of oral mucosal lesions is largely valueless except as a research tool. Cytology cannot be depended upon to give a reliable diagnosis in such a serious disorder or in pre-cancerous lesions.

Skin tumours

Skin consists of a superficial epidermis supported by a fibrovascular dermis. Melanocytes are pigment-producing cells that control skin pigmentation. All cells have the potential to become malignant. The most important predisposing factor for this is exposure to sunlight. Skin tumours include:

- epidermal tumours – basal-cell carcinoma (BCC) and squamous-cell carcinoma (SCC);

- malignant melanoma;
- non-melanocytic pigmented lesions;
- rare tumours.

Epidermal tumours

These are known to arise following prolonged exposure to ultraviolet light, and there is a strong association between lip cancer and exposure to sunlight. They are therefore usually found in sun-exposed skin (e.g. face, scalp and lower lip), particularly in elderly male patients who have lived or worked outdoors for many years. Fair-skinned individuals who have lived close to the equator are also at increased risk. For example, the incidence in Australia has been found to be about 20 times higher than that in the UK. Tobacco exposure, particularly from pipe smoking, is another recognized risk factor for lip cancer, perhaps due to thermal irritation from the pipe stem. Lip cancer is rare in AfroCaribbeans and Asians, who are protected by natural pigment, and in women who work outdoors less and perhaps have further skin protection provided by cosmetics.

Other less common aetiological factors are previous irradiation, xeroderma pigmentosum, albinism, arsenic ingestion and immunosuppression (e.g. following transplantation). BCCs may sometimes be part of a syndrome known as Gorling Goltz, which consists of multiple recurrent BCCs and recurrent multiple odontogenic keratocysts.

Potentially malignant conditions include solar keratosis, which presents as a raised, scaly erythematous lesion, sometimes with marked hyperkeratosis. Bowen's disease develops as a chronic, nodular, crusted or ulcerated plaque, which may be associated with sun-damaged skin.

BASAL-CELL CARCINOMA (RODENT ULCERS)

These vary considerably in appearance (nodular, ulcerated, cystic, pigmented or atrophic), and pigmented BCCs may occasionally be confused with melanoma. They should always be considered in any skin lesion which is not characteristic of any other condition. BCCs are generally slow-growing, and may take several years to reach 1 cm in diameter. Although growth is slow, they infiltrate into adjacent structures, making cosmetically satisfactory treatment difficult in the canthal region or the base of the nose. BCCs very rarely metastasize, but can cause extensive local destruction if neglected or incompletely excised.

SQUAMOUS-CELL CARCINOMA

These arise in sun-damaged skin and tend to present as an 'ulcer' which has failed to heal. Differentiation between SCCs and BCCs can sometimes be difficult. SCCs tend to be more aggressive than BCCs and, if left untreated, can metastasize to cervical nodes. Once this has occurred, the prognosis is considerably poorer.

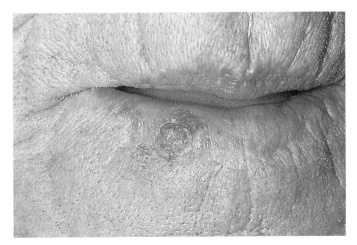

Figure 12.12 Squamous-cell carcinoma of the lower lip. Carcinoma in this site is strongly associated with chronic exposure to sunlight.

Both tumours can be treated satisfactorily with surgery or radiotherapy. In general, for lesions less than 1 cm in diameter surgery is easier, quicker, can be carried out under local anaesthesia and, with good local flap design, making use of lax skin and normal skin creases (see Fig. 4.2), excellent cosmetic results can be obtained (Fig. 12.13). If BCCs have a clearly defined margin

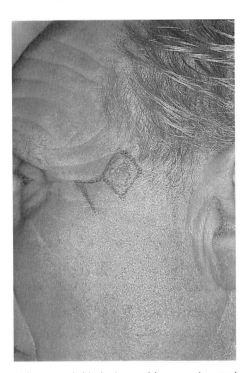

Figure 12.13 Rhomboid flap. Local skin laxity enables resections to be reconstructed using neighbouring tissue. Many different designs of flap exist.

they can be excised with a small cuff (1–2 mm) of normal tissue. However, the specimens must be clearly orientated and labelled in case excision is incomplete and further surgery is required. Alternatively, in cases where wide clearance is not possible (e.g. in the medial canthus of the eye), a frozen section can be made at the time of surgery to establish whether clearance has been achieved.

For larger lesions over 2 cm in diameter surgery is also preferred, since the tumour bulk makes cure by radiotherapy less predictable. Incisional biopsy is essential beforehand to confirm the diagnosis.

Reconstruction depends on the size of the defect. In general, the majority of BCCs in the UK present early, and reconstruction can be carried out either by simple closure of the wound, by local skin flaps, or by full-thickness skin grafts (Wolf grafts).

BCCs are said not to metastasize, although there are case reports in the literature of metastasis to cervical nodes and even to the liver. Small, well-differentiated SCCs seldom spread to lymph nodes. However, careful follow-up is necessary for larger, poorly differentiated tumours.

Non-melanocytic pigmented skin lesions

These lesions are important in that they may be confused with melanoma. They include basal cell papilloma, basal cell carcinoma, naevus, haemangioma, histiocytoma and pyogenic granuloma. In many cases excision biopsy with local flap closure is necessary to make the diagnosis.

Rare skin tumours

These include tumours arising from hair follicles, sweat glands and sebaceous glands. Most of these resemble and behave like low-grade BCCs, although some are more benign and a few may be more malignant.

Naevi and malignant melanoma (Fig. 12.14)

Common naevi and melanomas arise from melanocytes, i.e. the pigment-producing cells derived from the neural crest. Various benign pigmented lesions can develop, including freckle, lentigo, junctional naevus, compound naevus and blue naevus. Malignant melanoma is a malignant neoplasm of melanocytes. Like the epidermal tumours it is usually seen in fair-skinned people who live close to the equator. Important risk factors include the following:

- exposure to ultraviolet light, particularly in childhood;
- a high total number of naevi;
- a tendency to freckle;
- a family history of malignant melanoma.

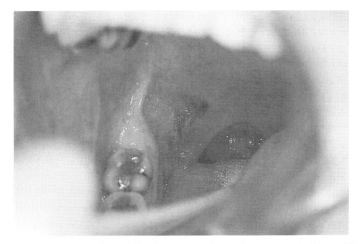

Figure 12.14 This pigmented patch in the retromolar region was an incidental finding during a routine dental check-up. Biopsy confirmed that this was a malignant melanoma.

The difficulty lies in deciding which naevi should be removed and which can be safely left. Indications for removal of naevi include a history of change, particularly bleeding, ulceration, 'satellite' nodules, irregular margin, variegate appearance (i.e. different shades of different colours) and itching. Because appearances vary considerably, melanoma must be considered in all pigmented skin lesions (and in some non-pigmented skin lesions). Ideally, suspicious naevi should be excised with a margin of 2–3 mm. However, incision biopsy may be performed when this would cause a large cosmetic defect.

Malignant melanomas are generally classified into four types:

- superficial spreading melanoma;
- nodular melanoma;
- lentigo maligna melanoma – this occurs particularly in sun-damaged skin, and is most commonly seen in the elderly, usually on the face, and occasionally on the neck or the backs of the hands and arms. It generally has a slow growth pattern and commonly occurs in a pre-invasive form, namely lentigo maligna or Hutchison's melanotic freckle;
- acral lentiginous melanoma involving the soles of the feet, palms of the hands or the nail beds.

Rare types of malignant melanoma include mucosal melanoma, which has been described in the nose, sinuses, mouth, eye and gastrointestinal tract. Occasionally there is a familial incidence of melanoma characterized by a distinctive type of larger mole that is present in large numbers – the dysplastic naevus syndrome.

Various staging systems have been developed to assess the prognosis. Melanoma can be divided into three stages:

- localized;
- regional spread (skin or lymph nodes);
- distant metastasis.

The depth of invasion can be classified according to 'Clark's levels', of which there are five, with level 1 corresponding to the best prognosis and level 5 to the worst. Alternatively, the maximum or 'Breslow' thickness may be used, which is also a good indicator of prognosis.

When surgery is considered, the site and size of the tumour and the age and general health of the patient need to be taken into account. Curative treatment ideally involves wide local excision in order to reduce the risk of local recurrence. Proximity to the nose, eye or mouth may occasionally prevent this ideal clearance. A 1-cm clearance should be regarded as a minimum. Most facial defects can be closed with local flaps, but if they are extensive, free flaps may be necessary.

Neck dissection in clinically normal necks may be undertaken depending on these factors, but is a controversial issue. Clinically positive or highly suspicious nodes should be excised by block and radical dissection.

Chemotherapy, immunotherapy and radiation therapy have generally been disappointing. Recently, interferons and interleukins have been tried, but at present they are currently only being used in clinical trials. Palliative radiotherapy is useful for the treatment of pain due to bone metastasis, but has little role to play in the primary treatment of the disease.

Kaposi's sarcoma

This typically occurs in elderly, Jewish males, most commonly as multiple nodules on the lower legs. However, it can present as a pigmented intra-oral lesion, particularly on the palate. Kaposi's sarcoma may be associated with immunosuppressive drugs or form part of the acquired immunodeficiency syndrome, where it may be the presenting sign. Treatment is usually with radiotherapy or chemotherapy if disseminated. Any underlying immunosuppression must also be taken into account.

Ameloblastoma

This is a tumour arising from 'odontogenic' epithelium, i.e. epithelium which would normally take part in tooth formation. Several subtypes exist.

Ameloblastomas account for about 1 per cent of all oral tumours, but are the commonest tumours to arise within the jaws (Fig. 12.15). The majority occur in the mandible, in the third molar region or ramus. Rarely they can develop in the adjacent soft tissues. They are benign but locally aggressive tumours which tend to recur locally following excision. This is particularly important in the case of maxillary tumours, where extension to the skull base and associated major vessels makes them potentially lethal.

Patients usually present with a painless hard swelling, or the tumour is a chance finding on an X-ray. Metastases are rare, but have been reported in the lung, lymph nodes and skull. Treatment depends on the site and type of

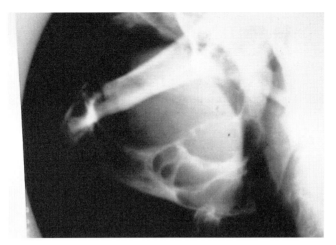

Figure 12.15 Ameloblastoma arising in an edentulous mandible. A tumour of this size can present as a swelling or with fracture of the jaw following a minor injury.

tumour. Wide resection is usually necessary, which in the maxilla involves a maxillectomy. With smaller mandibular tumours it may be possible to preserve the lower border of the bone and therefore retain facial contour. Postoperative radiotherapy may slow further growth, but should be regarded as palliative treatment only.

13 Surgical diseases of the salivary glands

Michael Perry

Management of clinically benign tumours
Management of clinically malignant tumours
Calculi (stones) and strictures
Infections of the salivary glands
Cysts of the salivary glands
Other diseases of the salivary glands

Saliva is produced by:

- *major salivary glands* – parotid, submandibular and sublingual;
- *minor salivary glands* – these line the mouth, palate and lips, and can occasionally be found in the nose.

Any of these glands can undergo malignant change.

The incidence of tumours of the salivary glands in the UK is approximately 3 to 4 per 100 000, although world-wide this varies from around 0.3 to 4 per 100 000. These tumours are slightly more common in females. Both benign and malignant tumours can occur at any age, although they are more commonly seen in middle-aged and elderly patients. Although they are more common in atomic-bomb survivors and in patients who have previously received irradiation of the neck, unlike oral cancer there are no other proven carcinogenic factors such as smoking.

The World Health Organization (WHO) has produced an extensive classification of salivary gland tumours, and currently there are over 40 different tumour types. The commonest tumour in the parotid gland is the benign pleomorphic adenoma. The muco-epidermoid tumour is the most common malignant salivary gland tumour (Fig. 13.1).

Patients may present with the following clinical features:

- swelling;
- pain;
- facial weakness (parotid gland);
- skin changes;

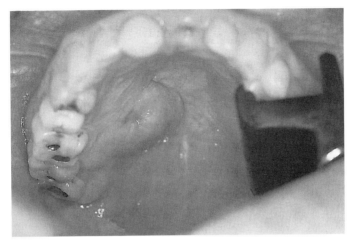

Figure 13.1 A muco-epidermoid tumour arising from salivary tissue in the hard palate. Swellings of this size usually require an incisional biopsy to be carried out prior to definitive treatment.

- poor hearing or earache;
- incidental finding.

Most parotid tumours present as painless, localized swellings which have been present for several months, although occasionally they may have been present for many years. Pain suggests infection or a rapidly growing malignant tumour. Other features suggestive of malignancy include facial nerve weakness, tethering of the lump, and rapid growth. Investigations vary from one unit to another and may include imaging, most commonly a CT scan or MRI scan. Fine-needle aspirate cytology is often undertaken, but its value is the subject of much debate. Some surgeons now take the view that none of these investigations significantly affects the management of such tumours, and may opt to remove the gland on clinical grounds only.

Tumours of the submandibular gland represent approximately 10 per cent of salivary gland tumours. Around two-thirds of these are pleomorphic adenomas, the remainder being malignant.

Tumours of the minor salivary glands represent about 10 per cent of salivary tumours and usually occur in the palate and upper lip; 45 per cent of these tumours are malignant. Swellings in the upper lip and hard palate should therefore always raise suspicions of a salivary gland neoplasm, and will nearly always require a biopsy.

Not all swellings of the major salivary glands are due to salivary tumours. Tumours can also arise from associated blood vessels, nerves, fat and lymphatic tissue. 'Tumour-like' conditions presenting as swellings include sarcoid, toxoplasmosis and sialosis. The latter is a painless swelling which may be associated with alcoholic cirrhosis, diabetes, acromegaly or bulimia.

Management of clinically benign tumours

The aim of treatment is complete excision without damage to associated structures such as:

• the parotid gland – facial nerve;
• the submandibular gland – mandibular branch of the facial nerve, lingual and hypoglossal nerves;
• the sublingual gland – lingual and hypoglossal nerves.

Parotid surgery

Tumours most commonly arise in the superficial lobe, i.e. superficial to the facial nerve which passes through the gland. These are usually removed with the whole lobe in order to ensure adequate clearance. The facial nerve is identified and all gland superficial to it is meticulously dissected off. With deeper tumours the whole gland is removed, leaving the nerve behind.

Pleomorphic adenomas are particularly prone to recur, which is why they are removed with such a large cuff of normal tissue. Recurrence may occur as long as 20 to 30 years after excision. Repeated operations carry an increasing risk of permanent facial weakness, but further surgery may be necessary with recurrent lumps, as there is a risk of malignant change occurring in long-standing pleomorphic adenomas.

Submandibular/sublingual surgery

The whole gland is usually removed. Submandibular glands are approached through a low incision in the neck, to avoid the mandibular branch of the facial nerve, whilst sublingual glands are taken out through the mouth.

Minor salivary tumours

These are usually excised with closure of the defect. Small tumours arising on the palate can be removed and the defect left 'raw' to heal or a dressing plate provided as with other tumours. With larger tumours, CT scans are often necessary to determine whether the tumour has eroded into the palate and floor of the nose, prior to excision. Most small tumours can be excised under local anaesthesia or as a day case.

Management of clinically malignant tumours

If possible, an attempt should be made to excise parotid tumours with preservation of the facial nerve. Depending on the type of tumour and its size, treatment may involve:

- excision of the gland;
- excision of the gland with involved adjacent tissue/neck dissection. As with oral cancers, reconstruction using local or free flaps may be necessary. If the facial nerve has to be sacrificed, a nerve graft can be used to 'bridge' the defect (see Chapter 4). Palatal defects can be closed with obturators or flaps;
- chemotherapy/immunotherapy/radiotherapy (e.g. lymphoma);
- radical surgery followed by adjuvant radiotherapy.

Following parotid surgery a small drain is usually placed prior to closure. Some surgeons place a pressure dressing for 24 h. Drains are usually removed the next day, and very often the patient can go home. Weakness of the facial nerve may occasionally be seen and is usually temporary. However, it is important that if the eyelids cannot protect the eye, a patch is placed and artificial tears or chlormycetin ointment prescribed until they can do so. In cases of marked weakness, where this is likely to persist for some time, the outer thirds of the eyelids can be sutured together – a lateral tarsorraphy. This helps to protect the eye and keep its surface lubricated with tears. Sutures are removed after 5 days.

Complications following parotid surgery

These include:

- facial weakness;
- salivary fistula (these often close spontaneously, although salivary suppressants may be prescribed);
- Frey's syndrome (sweating on eating) – this is thought to develop as a result of abnormal nerve connections between the gland and its overlying sweat glands;
- numb ear-lobe (division of great auricular nerve);
- wound breakdown;
- painful neuroma of the great auricular nerve.

Excision of the sublingual and submandibular glands is usually straightforward. Bleeding and haematoma formation are rare but important complications in view of the threat that they pose to the airway. Following excision of the sublingual gland the patient can eat a soft diet the following day. However, the floor of the mouth heals rapidly and a normal diet can soon be resumed. Good oral hygiene is important.

Calculi (stones) and strictures

Most calculi occur in the submandibular gland and duct, although they also commonly occur in the parotid gland. Calculi in the other salivary glands are rare. Strictures may arise from trauma, e.g. from cheek biting, dentures, following surgery or a previous calculus. Both conditions result in obstruction. Patients therefore usually complain of the following:

- recurrent or persistent swelling, especially at mealtimes;
- pain;
- symptoms relieved by discharge of saliva or pus from duct.

If saliva is allowed to stagnate in the gland, infection may develop (see below). Long-term obstruction leads to permanent glandular destruction.

Treatment

Depending on the type of obstruction, the site and the presence of glandular destruction, this may include:

- dilation of stricture;
- removal of calculus;
- reconstruction of duct;
- re-siting of duct;
- excision of gland.

Infections of the salivary glands

Both the major and minor salivary glands can become infected. 'Ascending' infection (i.e. bacteria in the saliva passing back up the ducts to the glands) commonly involves the parotid and submandibular glands. In such cases predisposing conditions may be associated (e.g. dehydration, diabetes mellitus, immunosuppression or pre-existing gland disease such as obstruction from either a calculus or a stricture). Fibrosis following radiotherapy may also predispose to infection.

Common clinical features

These include the following:

- fever;
- pain;
- erythema;
- tender swelling;
- discharge of pus from the duct;
- dry mouth;
- dehydration.

If infection is not treated early on this may develop into chronic or recurrent infection. Progressive destruction occurs which aggravates the situation, resulting in a non-functional gland.

Treatment

In the absence of an obvious abscess which requires incision and drainage, treatment initially consists of antibiotics, rehydration, analgesia and correction of any systemic conditions (e.g. diabetes). If an obstruction is found (e.g. a calculus or stricture) this needs to be removed to enable drainage. Gland massage, especially after meals, and 'lemon drops' to stimulate salivary flow help to maintain a flushing effect and prevent stagnation of saliva. Abscesses need to be incised and drained on an urgent basis. If infection persists or continues to recur excision of the gland may be necessary.

Cysts of the salivary glands

'Retention' or 'extravasation' cysts are commonly seen in the cheek and lower lip. They occur following trauma, usually a bite to the minor salivary glands resulting in scarring and obstruction. Every now and then they burst, discharging the saliva, only to recur at a later date. A ranula is a similar cyst arising from the sublingual gland. A sialocoele may arise in a major salivary gland following obstruction or previous surgery. Treatment usually involves excision of the cyst and associated gland.

Other diseases of the salivary glands

A variety of autoimmune and degenerative conditions can involve the salivary and lacrimal glands. Many of these do not require surgery but occasionally surgery is carried out to establish a diagnosis, or to remove painful/unsightly glands. Recurrent infection in a non-functioning gland is also an indication for removal. Sjögren's disease carries a risk of lymphomatous change, and removal may be required to establish this. Biopsy of minor salivary glands can usually be performed under local anaesthesia. More extensive surgery for open biopsy or excision of major salivary or lacrimal glands requires a general anaesthetic.

Patients may present with any of the following:

- xerostomia;
- swelling of the salivary gland or lacrimal gland;
- 'burning mouth';
- keratoconjunctivitis sicca;
- cosmetic deformity.

14 Orthognathic surgery and the temporomandibular joint (TMJ)

Michael Perry and Christine van der Valk

Over the last 30 years, orthognathic surgery has assumed an important role in oral and maxillofacial surgery. This is concerned with the correction of 'dentofacial' deformity, i.e. deformity involving the teeth, their supporting 'alveolar' bone and the jaws themselves (the mandible and maxillae). Case selection, assessment, treatment options and post-operative care will be described in this chapter.

Any malocclusion should not be considered in isolation during treatment planning, but *in conjunction with the face as a whole*. In many instances surgery to other parts of the face may be necessary in order to obtain the best results.

Facial growth follows a generally predictable pattern that usually results in a well-proportioned and almost symmetrical appearance. Deviations in growth may result in an appearance which to some may be unacceptable. Functional problems, particularly involving the bite (Fig. 14.1), speech, swallowing or the temporomandibular joint (TMJ) may also be associated with such deviations. These problems are due to the relative positions of the upper and lower jaws with respect to each other and the remainder of the face. Since the jaws support the teeth (dental arches), dental malpositions may also contribute significantly to the overall appearance. Therefore surgery in selected

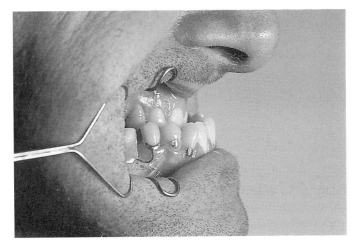

Figure 14.1   A gross 'Class III' malocclusion with significant functional and obvious aesthetic problems.

cases can result in functional and often marked aesthetic changes which can benefit the patient both physically and psychologically. However, it must be stressed that patients who undergo orthognathic surgery are not psychologically abnormal.

During facial growth and development of the occlusion (bite), the upper and lower teeth erupt into the 'best fit' possible. Where the supporting bones (skeletal bases) are only slightly abnormal, the teeth can adapt their position and compensate for this. This is known as 'dental compensation'. However, when the malposition of the jaws is more severe, this is not possible and an abnormal bite (malocclusion) develops. Depending on the bite, this can put the teeth at risk of injury or progressive 'gum disease'.

The initial position of the teeth and their position following orthodontics are important when deciding on treatment options. Simply to reposition the jaws without considering tooth position and angulation will result in a poor appearance that will probably relapse. Good results can therefore only be achieved with close co-operation between the orthodontist and the oral and maxillofacial surgeon during all stages of treatment. This is supported by a multidisciplinary team that includes maxillofacial technicians, oral hygienists and experienced nursing staff.

Types of deformity

Every case is unique, but patients can be broadly classified into those with:

- maxillary excess or deficiency;
- mandibular excess or deficiency (these must be considered in all three dimensions, i.e. facial profile, width and height);
- facial asymmetry;
- malocclusion which cannot be treated by orthodontics alone.

In addition, abnormalities of the following may be associated with the deformity:

- growth and development of the TMJ;
- chin;
- coronoid process;
- zygoma (cheek);
- orbit;
- nose;
- soft tissues (ears, nose, etc.).

Since the majority of cases are due to variations in growth, most are usually left until the patient's face is fully grown. To reposition the bones before then will produce unstable results as further growth alters the final appearance. However, where there is gross deformity leading to significant functional problems or psychological distress, surgery may be carried out earlier. This may be necessary in some cases of unilateral hypoplasia of the mandible (e.g. first-arch syndrome, or following trauma or infection), where reduced mandibular growth prevents the maxilla from developing on the same side. Early surgery enables the mandible to grow and allows normal maxillary development. However, further surgery may be necessary when the patient is fully grown.

Indications for treatment

Functional indications include the following:

- difficulties in chewing;
- difficulties with speech;
- reduced jaw movement;
- TMJ dysfunction;
- lip incompetence (inability to bring the lips together to protect the upper teeth);
- gum disease as a result of poorly aligned teeth;
- to help retain dentures;
- respiratory problems (e.g. sleep apnoea).

Aesthetic indications include the following:

- unacceptable appearance that causes the patient significant psychological distress.

Principles of assessment

History

Thorough assessment is essential. The reasons for seeking treatment must be established (is it the patient, parent, spouse or dentist who noted the abnormality?). Fortunately, very few medical conditions preclude surgery or the wearing of orthodontic appliances ('braces'). However, patients with uncontrolled epilepsy, congenital cardiovascular disease, some blood disorders and severe mental/physical handicap present particular problems and require careful assessment. Occasionally, children are seen whose general growth is unusual for their age. In most patients this is usually familial, although extreme variations may indicate unrecognized conditions such as acromegaly. Craniofacial deformity (see Chapter 17) is usually identified in infancy or early childhood. However, late presentation still occurs, or further treatment may be required. Patients with repaired clefts of the palate also frequently require orthognathic surgery.

The attitudes and expectations of both the patient and their parents or partner must be assessed. Treatment is often prolonged, requiring frequent visits to the orthodontist as well as the surgeon, and both must be fully aware of what this involves. A social history is therefore very important (time available to attend, distance to travel, whether the patient can afford time off work). It is also important to identify those patients or parents with unrealistic expectations, i.e. those who blame all of their difficulties (relationship, career and financial problems) on their appearance.

Examination

EXTRA-ORAL EXAMINATION

Clinical examination is one of the most important aspects of the evaluation, supplemented by special radiographs (cephalometrics) (Fig. 14.2). An assessment in all three dimensions, paying particular attention to the facial profile (mandibular/maxillary protrusion/retrusion), vertical proportions and symmetry of the face, is made (see Box 14.1). This includes both skeletal and 'soft' tissue features such as tongue and lip activity which can have an effect on tooth position. Inapppropriate correction of one without appreciating the effects of the other will be unaesthetic and lead to relapse.

BOX 14.1   Facial assessment – desirable features

- Symmetry
- Facial profile – the nose, lips and chin should take the shape of cupid's bow
- The upper, middle and lower thirds of the face should all be of equal height
- The intercanthal distance should be equal to that of the base of the nose
- The ears should be at the same level (mid-third of the face)
- The lips should be one-third of the distance between the base of the nose and the chin
- The corners of the mouth should be in line with the pupils

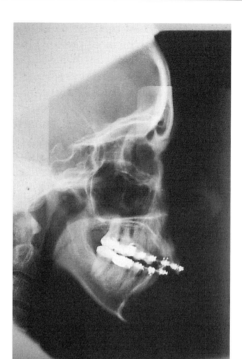

Figure 14.2 Lateral cephalogram. This enables the bony and dental contribution to the patient's appearance to be evaluated. The angles and measurements taken can be compared with 'normal' values for the general population.

INTRA-ORAL EXAMINATION

The teeth, gingiva (gums) and oral hygiene are examined to determine the need for planned extractions. *Orthodontics and surgery should not be undertaken in a patient with persistently poor oral hygiene.* The inclination of the teeth, shape of the dental arches and occlusion (?compensation) should be assessed.

Further assessment

To aid the examination, laboratory-produced 'study models' (Fig. 14.3) of the teeth and specific radiographs called cephalometrics are usually necessary. These can be used to measure various distances or angles of the bones/teeth, etc., which can then be compared to 'average' values for specific racial groups. This should confirm the clinical impression, i.e. what needs to be moved and by how much. Other investigations, such as bone scans, may be used if it is unclear whether the patient has stopped growing.

Prior to surgery, the patient should ideally be seen and assessed by a

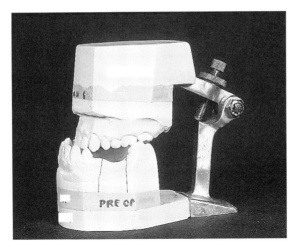

Figure 14.3 Study models. These enable detailed analysis of the patient's occlusion and also model 'surgery' to be carried out. Alternative osteotomies can be evaluated prior to 'the real thing'.

dietitian and speech and language therapist, and given instructions in oral hygiene by a hygienist. Immediately after surgery they will be unable to eat solid food, swallow normally or keep their mouth very clean. Nutrition and hygiene are important factors for ensuring a good recovery.

Treatment

Pre-surgical orthodontics

In most cases orthodontics to 'decompensate' the teeth is necessary. The aim is to 'align and co-ordinate' the dental arches into compatible shapes. Extractions (often third molars) can also be carried out. Fixed ('brace') or removable ('plate') appliances are available to move the teeth. 'Co-ordination' refers to positioning the upper and lower teeth so that *following* surgery they are in the desired positions with respect to each other. This simplifies the type of surgery required.

Surgical procedures

Over the years numerous techniques have been developed, each with its own advantages and drawbacks. It is not the purpose of this chapter to enter into the details of each procedure, but rather to outline the different types that are commonly in use. The options include osteotomies, ostectomies, onlays and inlays. Bone grafts may also be necessary.

BOX 14.2   Osteotomies and ostectomies

1 *Mandibular osteotomies*
- Ramus procedures – intra-oral, e.g. sagittal split, vertical sub-sigmoid
                            – extra-oral, e.g. inverted L, vertical sub-sigmoid
- Body procedures (e.g. ostectomy)
- Subapical or segmental
- Genioplasty

2 *Maxillary osteotomies*
- Le Fort I, Le Fort II, Le Fort III
- Segmental procedures (anterior or posterior)
- Palatal expansion
- Subapical

COMMON TECHNIQUES FOR THE MANDIBLE

Many different procedures are available for the lower jaw, although the vast majority of deformities can be corrected by only a few of these techniques. The choice is often down to the preference of the surgeon. No single technique is universally applicable.

Bilateral sagittal split osteotomy (BSSO) (Fig. 14.4)

This commonly used method enables the entire body of the mandible to be repositioned relative to the maxilla. It is especially useful where there is mandibular prognathism, retrognathism, asymmetry or an anterior open bite. Surgery is carried out through the mouth, thus avoiding facial scars. Bone cuts are made on both sides, and the mandible is split in a controlled manner separating the outer (buccal) cortical plates from the inner (lingual) cortical

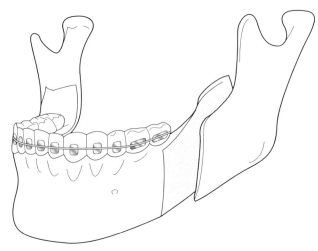

Figure 14.4 Sagittal split osteotomy.

plates. The mobile anterior segment carrying the teeth is then free to be repositioned, whilst maintaining the original position of the temporomandibular joint and chewing muscles. This method involves exposure of the inferior alveolar and lingual nerves, and therefore carries a small but real risk of injury with numbness to the lower lip and tongue. Post-operatively the patient can eat soft food and drink the next day.

Ramus osteotomies

Here the vertical ramus is cut in order to reposition the anterior body and teeth. This can be carried out through the mouth or extra-orally. This is useful for closure of anterior open bites. Fixation using miniplates or IMF and bone grafts may be required. Again the lingual and inferior alveolar nerves are at risk.

Body ostectomy

This can be used to reduce an abnormally long mandibular body, close an anterior open bite or correct asymmetry. Cuts are placed between the roots of the teeth in the horizontal body, so that the anterior fragment can be moved. These are made through the mouth. Where the fragment is moved forwards, blocks of bone (usually iliac crest) are inserted into the gaps created and fixed with wires or miniplates. This is not as stable as with sagittal splits, and patients often require some form of intermaxillary fixation postoperatively.

Post-condylar grafts

In some cases of mandibular retrognathism, blocks of cartilage can be used to reposition the entire jaw forward. Both temperomandibular joints are approached through incisions placed just in front of the ear. Cartilage is fixed to the root of the zygomatic arch between the head of the condyle and the bony auditory meatus. Only relatively small forward movements are possible.

COMMON TECHNIQUES FOR THE MAXILLA

Le Fort osteotomies

The maxilla can be osteotomized at several levels corresponding to the 'Le Fort' fracture classification, although modifications exist. The commonest osteotomy is at the Le Fort I level, i.e. effectively cutting above the roots of the teeth, supporting bone and palate. These are 'pedicled' on the adjacent mucosa and soft palate from which they receive their blood supply. The mobile segment can then be repositioned in any direction and held in position using miniplates or wires. Bone grafting, commonly from the iliac crest, may be needed for certain movements.

Segmental osteotomies

These are used when a *localized* abnormality of the bite exists, or as a compromise when the patient is unwilling to undergo more extensive surgery.

Protrusion of the upper/lower anterior teeth may be corrected by osteotomizing the proclined segment, which is then repositioned.

BIMAXILLARY OSTEOTOMY

This term is slightly confusing but refers to osteotomies of both the maxilla and the mandible in the same patient. Correction of both jaws may be necessary in order to obtain the best facial profile, rather than simply moving one to obtain the desired bite. The commonest combination is the Le Fort I osteotomy and bilateral sagittal splitting osteotomy (BSSO).

SURGERY TO THE CHIN

A small chin is often associated with a retruded or small lower jaw. However, it is important to distinguish between these as the treatment for each is different. Where significant retrognathism is present, a mandibular osteotomy (see above) is required. Where *only* the chin is small, correction may be possible using an onlay (see below) or genioplasty.

Genioplasty (Fig. 14.5)

This involves isolating the chin from the mandible, which can then be repositioned. Surgery is performed through the mouth, and the bone is cut below the roots of the teeth and mental nerve. The nerve is at risk of injury where it leaves the mandible to enter the lower lip. This can result in permanent numbness. The chin can be moved forwards, backwards, rotated, or its height altered. Any gaps are filled with bone, cartilage or synthetic material. The new position is held with miniplates, wires or screws.

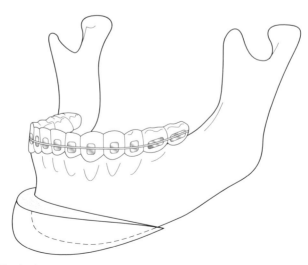

Figure 14.5 Genioplasty.

CONDYLAR HYPERPLASIA

'Developmental hyperplasia', or overgrowth of the mandibular condyle, can result in overgrowth of the affected side and asymmetry. Secondary deformity in the maxilla can occur with development of an abnormal bite. Early treatment of the affected condyle as soon as possible may restore normal growth and improve symmetry. The options include a 'high condylar shave' (intracapsular condylar reduction) or condylectomy, with or without replacement of the condyle. By 6–12 months after excision, a new condyle will have regenerated. If the deformity is not diagnosed until late, a mandibular osteotomy on the affected side may be necessary.

MANDIBULAR HEMIHYPERTROPHY

This results in lowering of the occlusal plane on the affected side, with downgrowth of the lower border of the mandible. Secondary deformity of the maxilla may occur. The deformity is predominantly in the vertical plane, and usually the midlines of the upper and lower dental arches remain coincident. Correction of this may require removal of excess bone from the lower border of the mandible, or if the occlusion is severely disrupted, a two-jaw procedure.

CORONOID HYPERPLASIA

The temporalis muscle is attached to the coronoid process and is one of the 'muscles of mastication' needed for chewing. Elongation of the coronoid process can result in limitation of mouth-opening due to impingement against the zygomatic arch under which the temporalis tendon passes. The cause of this is unknown. In severe cases one or both coronoid processes can be excised through an intra-oral approach.

Onlays

An onlay is a non-resorbable material that is placed on the surface of a bone in order to improve its contour. Various types exist, including:

- autografts (taken from the patient);
- homografts (taken from another human);
- zenografts (taken from another animal);
- allografts (manufactured).

Autografts

These are common in the UK, and are usually composed of bone or cartilage. Donor sites include iliac crest, rib and calvarium (bone) or rib, ear and nasal septum (cartilage). These are particularly useful in the chin and cheek areas as an alternative to osteotomies for minor defects. They can also be used to fill in bony contours (e.g. lower border of the mandible and skull). Usually they are placed via the mouth. However, pressure from the overlying soft tissues may lead to underlying bone resorption (Wolf's law) if it is too high. Grafts are secured with miniplates, wires, screws or tissue adhesives.

Allografts

Many synthetic materials are available as alternatives to natural materials. These include stainless steel, cobalt chrome, acrylic, teflon, silastic, nylon and hydroxyapatite. These do not undergo resorption, although pressure on the underlying bone can sometimes lead to its resorption if it is too high. All materials are at risk of infection or extrusion, and may have to be removed.

Fixation techniques (see Chapter 11)

The repositioned bone(s) need to be held securely in place until normal healing has occurred. It takes 3 to 4 weeks for the union to be strong enough to take significant loads, and the patient needs to be on a soft diet during this time.

BOX 14.3   Techniques available for bone fixation

- Intermaxillary fixation (IMF) (arch bars, eyelet wires, orthodontic brackets); splints and wafers may be necessary to improve the 'fit' of the teeth;
- Miniplates
- Screws (e.g. Lag or bicortical)
- External fixation (rare)

BOX 14.4   Complications of surgery

Severe complications are rare, but swelling and temporary numbness are relatively common. Other complications include:

- airway and respiratory complications (usually with IMF);
- haemorrhage;
- facial swelling;
- pain;
- medical complications of surgery and anaesthesia.

In the longer term, complications may include:
- numbness;
- non-union;
- relapse;
- difficulties in chewing, mouth opening and speech;
- TMJ dysfunction;
- sinusitis;
- nasal obstruction;
- patient dissatisfaction with outcome.

Post-operative care

Depending on the procedure and local practice, patients may return to the ward or spend the night in an ICU/HDU. During the early stages the most important complications to look out for are airway and respiratory problems, haemorrhage, severe facial swelling, pain and medical complications of surgery and anaesthesia. Constant monitoring of the airway is essential, particularly where the jaws have been wired together (IMF), as airway problems and poor respiratory function are more likely. Oozing of blood is common post-operatively, but should not be significant and should quickly settle. Since much of the bleeding is swallowed, careful observations and assessment of fluid balance are necessary. Steroids (e.g. dexamethasone) are often given on induction and then post-operatively to reduce the amount of swelling and discomfort. Pain is often less than might be expected for the degree of surgery. Regular non-steroidal anti-inflammatory or paracetamol-based drugs are usually sufficient, and opiates are rarely required after 24 h. Antibiotics are often required to reduce the risk of post-operative infection.

Most patients recover remarkably well and may be fit for discharge the next day (single-jaw osteotomy) or within 24–48 h (bimaxillary osteotomy). However, not all patients recover this quickly, and some may need to stay in hospital longer. Pain, swelling and difficulty in swallowing are the main reasons for delayed recovery. The lips are often swollen as a result of retraction during surgery. Vaseline or steroid-based ointments can help to reduce the swelling, especially if applied before or during surgery.

Post-operative care (the next day)

Radiographs are taken to check the initial post-operative position and fixation, and to ensure that there are no unrecognized complications (e.g. dislocated condyle, fractures). At this stage the maintenance of good oral hygiene is difficult, and most patients need help from a hygienist. Hygiene technique needs to be reinforced, supplemented by regular antiseptic (e.g. corsodyl) and hot salt-water mouthwashes. Patients are discharged when it is felt appropriate for them and it is known that they will receive the necessary care at home. The airway should be re-checked to ensure that there is no potential restriction and all bleeding has stopped. The patient must feel confident that he or she can cope properly at home with an adequate diet. Regular outpatient reviews must be arranged, especially in the early post-operative period.

Post-surgical orthodontics

Surgery alone rarely produces a perfect result, and othodontics is often required post-operatively to detail the occlusion (Fig. 14.6).

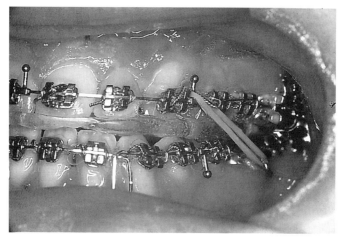

Figure 14.6 Post-operative orthodontics following bimaxillary osteotomy. Appropriately placed elastics aid the 'fine tuning' of the patient's occlusions. Plastic wafers are often used to guide the occlusion and aid stability until the osteotomy has healed.

The temporomandibular joint (TMJ)

BOX 14.5 Temporomandibular joint (TMJ) disorders

- TMJ pain dysfunction syndrome/internal derangement
- Osteoarthrosis/inflammatory/degenerative joint disease
- Infective arthritis
- Fractures/dislocation
- Ankylosis
- Condylar hyperplasia or hypoplasia
- Idiopathic condylar resorption

Introduction

TMJ pain is to the maxillofacial surgeon what low back pain is to the orthopaedic surgeon – common, often difficult to treat, not fully understood, and only a small proportion of cases need aggressive surgery. Indeed, both are often seen in the same patient. Symptoms that arise from the temporomandibular joint are common and include the following:

- pain;
- clicking;
- locking;
- limitation of mouth opening;
- stiffness.

Treatment aims to relieve pain and improve function. By far the most common condition is facial arthromyalgia, which is usually treated without surgery. Surgery to the TMJ should be regarded as a last resort (except in trauma and malignancy), to be used only after other measures have failed.

Temporomandibular joint pain dysfunction syndrome (facial arthromyalgia)

Temporomandibular joint pain dysfunction syndrome (TMJPDS) is a descriptive term that refers to pain arising from the temporomandibular joint and muscles of mastication. It is one of the commonest causes of facial pain after odontalgia.

The aetiology of TMJPDS is unknown, although stress, often associated with 'parafunctional habits' (e.g. bruxism) is a common feature. Occlusal disorders have been considered by some authorities, although this remains speculative.

Some evidence suggests that, in susceptible patients, changes in the biochemical environment of the temporomandibular joint result in a destructive arthropathy. For instance, symptomatic improvement in *non*-depressed patients has been described using tricyclic antidepressant drugs (nortryptyline). Enzyme deficiency (tyramine conjugase) has also been identified in these patients. However, the relationship between this and facial pain is unclear. Suggested mediators of the pain in facial arthralgia include the following:

- leukotrines (15-hydroxyeicosatetranoic acid);
- oxygen-derived free radicals;
- neuropeptides (e.g. substance P).

A significant number of patients respond well to reassurance or placebo treatment. Other measures include bite guards, analgesics, exercises, occlusal adjustment, intra-articular steroid injections, short-wave diathermy, ultrasound and laser therapy. Fluoxetine, a specific serotonin re-uptake inhibitor (SSRI), also appears to be effective.

Internal derangement

The Consensus Conference for Temporomandibular Surgery, at its meeting in Buenos Aires in 1992, defined internal derangement as 'a localized mechanical fault in the joint which interferes with its smooth action'. It may also occur in association with facial arthromyalgia. Surgery may be indicated for:

- failure of conservative treatment;
- clicking and locking of the joint.

Treatment includes:

- splint therapy;
- arthroscopic lavage;
- meniscopexy (meniscoplasty);
- menisectomy.

Osteoarthrosis (degenerative joint disease), rheumatoid arthritis and related autoimmune disease

Symptoms include:

- chronic pain;
- crepitus;
- difficulty in chewing;
- reduced mouth opening.

Treatment includes:

- anti-inflammatory analgesics with or without physical therapy;
- arthroscopic lavage;
- meniscopexy (meniscoplasty);
- condylectomy with or without replacement with a prosthesis;
- synovectomy (rheumatoid).

Rheumatoid arthritis of the temporomandibular joint

Rheumatoid arthritis involving the TMJ can result in granulation tissue proliferating on the articular surface, with subsequent joint destruction. Patients frequently complain of penetrating, aching pain and later joint restriction and ankylosis. Treatment includes heat application, joint physiotherapy, TENS, non-steroidal anti-inflammatory drugs (NSAIDs) and, when necessary, joint excision or reconstruction.

Infective arthritis

This is uncommon but potentially very severe, as infection may spread into the middle cranial fossa. Symptoms include:

- pyrexia;
- pain;
- swelling;
- erythema;
- suppuration;
- restricted mouth.

Management involves intravenous antibiotics and, if there is pus, incision and drainage. Occasionally, in cases of severe or recurrent infection, debridement (including condylectomy) may be necessary.

Ankylosis

Abnormal union across a joint space may be termed 'ankylosis'. This can be either fibrous or bony in origin. As a a result, patients experience restricted jaw movement, particularly mouth opening, affecting chewing and speech. Ankylosis in children can lead to restricted facial growth.

Depending on the cause, treatment may include:

- excision of the joint (gap arthroplasty);
- condylectomy and joint reconstruction using a costochondral graft;
- condylectomy and prosthesis;
- coronoidectomy;
- myotomy;
- conservative treatment to discourage reankylosis (biphosphonates, NSAIDs, physiotherapy).

Arthroscopy

Just as in orthopaedics, this involves the passage of a fine, rigid, fibre-optic scope into the joint space, enabling visualization of the articular surfaces. In expert hands a limited number of procedures may also be possible to remove pathology or reposition the meniscus. Success rates vary, but are generally very good so long as those cases that will benefit are identified correctly.

15 Aesthetic facial surgery

Michael Perry

Aesthetic surgery may be described as surgery carried out to improve or 'correct' the appearance of a patient. Very often the patient is not ill or does not have a disease as such for which surgery is necessary, although there are times when aesthetic techniques may be useful following trauma or surgery for cancer. Some of the more common problems will be described in this chapter.

It is essential that the surgeon deals with the problem as the patient sees it and not as they do. After all, the patient has to live with the final results and therefore must be satisfied with the outcome. During assessment, it is important to evaluate the patient's psychological profile and any expectations they may have of surgery. Although the majority of patients requesting aesthetic surgery are psychologically well adjusted, studies have shown that a significant number may have underlying psychiatric problems. For example, 'body morphoeic disorder' (or 'dysmorphobia') is a condition in which a minor physical 'defect' is believed by the patient to be noticeable to others, although his or her appearance is considered to be within normal limits. This may be associated with schizophrenia. In such cases consultation with a psychiatrist may be necessary. It is also important that the patient does not have unrealistic expectations of what will be achieved following treatment. Clear and honest discussion both before and after surgery is therefore essential, and both surgeon and patient must have a clear understanding of what surgery can offer.

Many techniques are available to 'improve' a patient's appearance, some of which have been discussed in previous chapters. Commonly used techniques include:

- baldness treatment;
- blepharoplasty;
- chemical exfoliation;
- chin augmentation and maxillary onlay;
- correction of masseteric hypertrophy;
- dermabrasion;
- face-lift and brow suspension;
- fat injection;
- gingival recontouring;
- laser surgery;

- lip enhancement;
- lipectomy;
- orbital decompression;
- orthognathic surgery;
- osseointegrated implants;
- pinnaplasty;
- rhinoplasty and septoplasty;
- scar revision.

Patient assessment

When assessing facial characteristics (e.g. nose, lips, cheeks, ears, etc.), it is important that these are viewed in the context of the face *as a whole* in order to produce an overall harmonious appearance. This is particularly subjective, and what may be appealing to one individual may be totally unacceptable to another. The patient's views are therefore essential, as the 'technically perfect' final aesthetic result may not be seen as such by the patient.

However, there are some guidelines based on facial proportions. This includes dividing the face into thirds and equal fifths in the vertical plane. Facial profile is also important, particularly when considering orthognathic surgery, although patients rarely see themselves in true profile.

Baldness (alopecia)

When an isolated patch of bald scalp is present (e.g. following a scalp burn), but the remainder of the hair is unaffected and of good quality, this may be managed with the use of tissue expansion (see Chapter 4). Alternatively, for male pattern baldness, hair transplantation may be carried out. This involves harvesting small 'plugs' of skin containing hairs and their follicles, which are then transplanted to the bald areas.

Blepharoplasty

'Bags' around the eyes are one of the earliest signs of ageing in the face. Occasionally these can be so severe as to interfere with vision. A history of conjunctivitis, styes and ocular herpes infection is important, as these may recur following surgery. Similarly, a history of dry eyes may contraindicate surgery, as any reduction in the protective function of the eyelids may aggravate the situation, resulting in corneal abrasions. The 'bags' are caused by various combinations of excess skin and fat and lax eyelid muscles, and the relative amounts of each must be determined before surgery. Surgery involves excising excess skin, 'debulking' any excess fat and repairing any weak muscles. Complications include haematoma, inadequate or excessive reduction, inability to close the lids properly, dry eyes, watering eyes and, rarely, blindness.

Chemical exfoliation (chemical peel)

This is a technique which is often used in the management of the 'ageing face', some pigmented patches and superficial acne scars. It involves the application of various 'wounding' agents, such as trichloracetic acid (TCA), 'Jessners' solution, alpha-hydroxy acids and phenol, to the skin in order to remove superficial lesions. Healing during the following months results in improved-quality skin, although there are limitations to this technique. By using different chemical agents different depths of peel can be achieved, and in some cases the procedure can be repeated if necessary after several months. Care and experience in the use of this technique are essential, as being predominantly acids the solutions can result in burns to the skin and eyes if they are not applied correctly. Other complications include phenol toxicity, scarring around the eyelids with ectropion and depigmentation.

Chin augmentation and malar implants

Improvement of the shape and projection of the chin can be carried out in several ways. For augmentation the choice is essentially between osteotomies (genioplasty; see Chapter 14) and onlays. Although placing onlays is technically easier, and can be carried out under local anaesthesia, complications may be associated with skin incisions and the materials used. With large augmentations, the pressure exerted by the skin may stimulate resorption of the underlying bone and change the profile. For minor augmentation, cartilage can be used which is taken from either the patient or an alternative source. Synthetic materials include silicone or proplast. The implant can be placed for either an intra-oral or extra-oral route. Although the intra-oral route avoids skin incisions, there is a higher rate of infection and displacement of the implant. Alternatively, external incisions could be placed with less risk of infection but with a resulting scar. Complications of implants include infection, migration, intra-oral exposure, bleeding and bone resorption.

In a similar way to the chin, augmentation of the cheeks (zygoma) can be carried out with implants or by osteotomizing and repositioning the bones. Silastic, proplast or hydroxyapatite implants can be used, these being placed either through the skin (blepharoplasty incision) or through the mouth.

Correction of masseter muscle hypertrophy

The masseter muscle is one of the powerful chewing muscles lying on the surface of the vertical portion or ramus of the mandible. Chronic hypertrophy of one or both masseter muscles can result in swelling of the lower part of the face, with asymmetry or excessive width. The cause of this is unknown, although it has been suggested that familial and acquired types exist. Jaw clenching, bruxism and the habit of chewing on one side have been suggested as contributing factors. The diagnosis is usually obvious in that the swelling is soft in the relaxed state but becomes quite solid on clenching the teeth. In the first instance, aggravating factors such as bruxism should be dealt with. Other treatments include muscle relaxants and tranquillizers, but these should be avoided in the long term. Botulinum toxin injected into the muscle is also very effective. This paralyses the muscle which then atrophies. Surgical correction is occasionally necessary, and involves resecting part of the muscle through the mouth.

Dermabrasion

This technique can be used as an adjunct to 'rejuvenation' surgery or in the management of superficial scars. In essence it involves mechanically removing the superficial layers of the skin using diamond burrs, wire brushes or some other method. The skin then heals by epithelial regeneration. So long as this process is not performed too deep, healing is complete, with no scarring and excellent results. However, dark-skinned patients should be cautioned about this technique, because it can result in hypo- or hyperpigmentation.

Fat injection

This may be used to 'smooth out' minor defects or hollows in the soft tissues where the underlying bones are normal. Fat is harvested from another site, such as the abdominal wall, by liposuction and is injected into the defect in order to distend the tissues. Care is needed as significant resorption can occur, and a degree of overcompensation may be necessary. The fat may also necrose and become infected if too much is used at a time.

Gingival contouring

This can be undertaken in patients whose gums are grossly enlarged but otherwise disease free. The commonest cause of gingival swelling is poor oral hygiene resulting in gingivitis. Here the swelling is reversible once hygiene is improved. However, in longstanding cases and as a side-effect of some drugs such as phenytoin and nifedipine, excessive growth can occur which may persist after withdrawal of the drug. Swelling around the necks of the teeth reduces the amount of tooth shown when smiling. In selected cases the gingiva may be trimmed back to expose the full length of the tooth crown, thereby improving the appearance of the smile. It is essential that any inflammation is treated prior to surgery.

Laser surgery

This is becoming increasingly popular in head and neck surgery, particularly in the field of aesthetics. Laser-resurfacing techniques are used as alternatives to blepharoplasty, face-lifts and other techniques to 'iron out' minor skin wrinkles. This effectively burns the superficial layers of the skin to a pre-set depth, after which healing occurs to produce a more satisfactory appearance. Carbon dioxide and Erbium:YAG lasers are used to produce a beam of the correct wavelength and penetration depth. When using lasers both patient and staff must be protected from potentially sight-threatening injuries, and protective goggles should always be worn.

Lip enhancement (vermilion advancement, collagen injection)

The vermilion is the visible red area of the lips, which is usually more prominent in females. When the lips are thin and the upper lip is long, advancement of the upper lip can be carried out to improve the amount of vermilion that is seen and, in selected cases, enhancement of the cupid's bow. A thin strip of skin is excised just above the vermilion border, which allows the remainder to be advanced to its new position. This involves an incision across the full width of the lip, and therefore suturing must be meticulous. Alternatively, bovine collagen may be injected to give the lips a fuller appearance. This has the advantage of not involving an incision, and the effect can be temporarily imitated beforehand by simply injecting sterile saline (which slowly resorbs) into the lip.

Lipectomy

This procedure is often carried out in the submental, submandibular and buccal fat regions, and in the nasolabial folds. With ageing, the skin becomes less elastic and fat is redistributed with recession around the orbits and temples and sagging in the submental and submandibular regions. Fat accumulates around the chin and jowls. Suction lipectomy involves a high-vacuum system which disrupts and aspirates fat globules via a variety of different-sized cannulas. Submental and submandibular lipectomy can be performed whenever there is excessive fat or a 'double chin' between the skin and the platysma muscle.

   Post-operatively an elasticated dressing is necessary to maintain uniform compression, prevent haematoma formation and encourage good soft tissue draping. This is necessary for up to 2–3 weeks. Complications include haematoma and bruising, persistent oedema, injury to the mandibular and cervical branches of the facial nerve, numbness and wrinkling, and scar tracks.

Orbital decompression for thyroid eye disease

Graves disease or autoimmune hyperthyroidism can affect the orbits in up to a third of cases, resulting in lid retraction, proptosis, difficulties in making eye movements and, if severe, corneal ulceration. This has been suggested to be due to the deposition of glycosaminoglycans in the orbital tissues, resulting in an increase in their overall volume. Even following treatment these problems may persist, and although often moderate, they can result in significant cosmetic and functional problems. Orbital decompression can be achieved by the removal of one or more of the bony orbital walls and incision of the periosteum. This allows some of the orbital fat to herniate through, thereby reducing the amount of tissue that is directly behind the eye. The procedure is not without significant risks, the most obvious one being blindness, and careful case selection is therefore essential.

Pinnaplasty (otoplasty, correction of 'bat' ears)

Excessive prominence of the ears is a relatively common problem which, particularly in children, can often lead to much ridicule. The prominence is due to the natural shape of the cartilage, which is highly elastic and difficult to mould, tending to return to its former shape after any pressure is released. In the very young (i.e. infants) some authorities believe that moulding is possible with appropriate dressings. However, it is generally accepted that this potential is rapidly lost and thereafter the only way to bring about permanent changes is by surgery. In such cases most authorities consider that surgery should not be carried out until the child is at least 5 years old.

Many techniques have been developed over the years. These involve either weakening the cartilage in 'key' areas so that it can be reshaped by sutures and dressings, or using non-resorbable sutures to hold the cartilage permanently in its desired shape. Skin is excised on the inner aspect of the pinna to help 'pin' it back. Common approaches include the 'Mustarde' and 'Anterior scoring' techniques. Of equal importance in the technique is the use of a well-conformed pressure dressing which needs to be worn up to 3 weeks after surgery. The aims of surgery are not to flatten the ears against the side of the head, but to reduce the degree of prominence and to achieve symmetry in projection. Complications include haematoma formation, chondritis, overcorrection, 'telephone' deformity, wound infection and relapse.

Rhinoplasty

Records of rhinoplasty date back to 2500BC in Egypt and India. Reconstruction of defects was carried out using skin from the forehead, cheeks and buttocks. Today surgery may be required for aesthetic reasons, following trauma, or in patients with cleft lip. The usual indications are as follows:

- to straighten a bent nose;
- to reduce a dorsal hump;
- to narrow a wide nose;
- to alter the nasal tip;
- a combination of the above.

Because of its prominent location, the nose significantly influences the overall appearance of the face, with associated psychological, sexual and cultural significance. It is often a focal point for patients who have concerns about their sexual identity, and among transsexuals rhinoplasty is often necessary for the success of a new female identity. Noses also reflect an individual's racial or ethnic origins (e.g. the high arching nose of the Asian or semitic individual and the flat nasal profile of the AfroCaribbean or oriental).

'Normal' noses vary considerably in size and shape between different individuals. A pleasing appearance depends in part on the relationship of the nose to the rest of the face; a nose that is considered to be attractive in one person may look unsightly in another.

The nose is essentially a pyramidal structure consisting of an underlying bone and cartilaginous skeleton over which the skin is draped. Skin quality varies considerably between individuals and in some medical conditions. Where it is thin, the underlying skeleton can be clearly defined. Associated facial muscles also contribute to the overall contour, and together they may aggravate or disguise changes in the underlying skeleton following surgery. The muscles arise from the adjacent maxilla and insert into the lower cartilages and skin.

Internally, the nose is divided by a vertical partition, the septum, that is composed of cartilage anteriorly and bone posteriorly. This provides some support and is important in nasal projection and the position of the nasal tip. From the side walls project the turbinate bones or conchi, which are covered by distensible mucosa. The function of these is to warm and moisten inspired air. Problems with either the septum or the turbinates can interfere with the passage of air and the drainage of the sinuses.

When considering the proportions of the nose, the basic shape is a trapezoid when viewed from the front, and an equilateral triangle when viewed from the 'worm's-eye' position. When viewed from the side, the apparent degree of projection is significantly affected by the dorsum which, if humped, gives the appearance of increased length. The nose is not a static structure, and the effects of facial movement, in particular smiling, should also be assessed.

OPERATIVE TECHNIQUE

Aesthetic surgery should ideally be carried out after the nose has fully grown (about 15 years in girls and 17 years in boys), as surgery before then may alter growth unfavourably. However, in severely deformed cases or where there is significant functional deformity, surgery before that time may be justified.

Rhinoplasties may be either 'closed' or 'open'.

Closed rhinoplasty involves performing surgery through small skin stab incisions placed alongside the nose, and through mucosal incisions which therefore cannot be seen. This approach is usually reserved for less complex cases, such as post-traumatic rhinoplasty requiring straightening only. Through these small incisions the skin may be dissected off the underlying bones and cartilage, and the bones can be osteostomized or refractured, enabling them to be repositioned. Irregular contours may also be smoothed and a prominent dorsal hump, if necessary, excised or smoothed.

Open rhinoplasty is carried out when good access to the underlying cartilage is required, and is therefore normally used for more complicated cases, such as 'cleft' noses. Incisions are placed around the base of the columella, extending into the nasal airways, and by careful dissection the skin may be peeled off or 'degloved' from the underlying cartilages to expose them fully. This enables more precise surgery to be carried out, depending on the desired results. Surgery may involve trimming of the alar cartilages or soft tissue, or some form of augmentation using cartilage obtained from elsewhere (e.g. the septum or ear).

During the surgical technique, good care of the tissues is essential. The skin and muscles are sensitive to post-operative swelling, and if stretched or damaged they can scar, with subsequent deformity.

Post-operatively, nasal splints are often applied to support the tissues and minimize the amount of post-operative oedema. Depending on the surgery, different forms of splints are available, ranging from adhesive tape (steri-strips) to mouldable splints or plaster of Paris casts. The choice of splint is determined by the surgeon's preference. Nasal packs are often required.

Complications include swelling and oedema, low-grade infection, skin disorders (e.g. allergy sensitivity, or skin pustules forming beneath a dressing, formation of telangiectasis and hypo- or hyperpigmentation) and unsatisfactory final appearance.

Septoplasty

This is often performed at the same time as the rhinoplasty, although deviation of the septum may sometimes be the only problem, with reduced air entry and deviation of the nasal tip. In essence, the lining over the nasal septum is stripped off on both sides of the cartilage, which is then repositioned in the midline. Simply repositioning the cartilage will not work, as it is elastic and will simply spring back once the nasal packs have been removed. Therefore a variety of techniques have been developed to enable permanent positioning, which may involve scoring the cartilage or removing portions of it. Once the cartilage has been repositioned, nasal packs are applied to prevent haematoma formation under the lining. These are often left in place for 24 h.

16 Pre-prosthetic surgery and osseo-integrated implants

Michael Perry

Pre-prosthetic surgery

Osseo-integrated implants

Over the years improvements in dental education and care have meant that fewer people are losing all of their teeth as a result of caries or gum disease. Many elderly people still have a full or nearly full set of teeth. However, teeth are still lost either due to dental neglect or as a result of injuries or cancer. This chapter will describe how dental rehabilitation may be improved or achieved with the use of adjunctive procedures and implants. Extra-oral implants are also becoming more important, as the quality of prostheses is now often better than that of reconstructive techniques.

Various options exist for replacing lost teeth, depending on how many and which ones are missing, the available skills, patient preference and cost. Prostheses (dentures) are a common choice which can be retained in the mouth either by learned muscle control and 'suction', or by anchoring them to the bone via implants.

After construction of a new set of dentures, the initial fit and patient satisfaction tend to diminish over the years, partly as a result of continuous resorption of the supporting alveolar bone. With progressively worsening fit of the denture, retention and stability decrease. The ability to adapt to these changes varies considerably between patients. However, for many individuals the reduced stability and retention result in pain, ulcers and difficulty in talking and eating. In severe cases this can eventually interfere with adequate nutritional intake and the ability to communicate with ease and confidence.

Bone resorption tends to affect the mandible more than the maxilla, and therefore patients usually complain about their lower denture. For many, a new set of well-fitting dentures will resolve the problems. However, surgery may be required to help to provide enough support and retention for the prosthesis. The aims are to enable the patient to chew their food efficiently and be free of discomfort. This is termed 'pre-prosthetic surgery'.

Pre-prosthetic surgery

Pre-prosthetic surgery is indicated in those patients who are unable to tolerate even a well-constructed denture due to unfavourable soft tissues or supporting bone. In addition to pain and functional problems, gross jaw disproportion (reducing denture retention) and an exaggerated gag reflex may mean that surgery is necessary.

Sometimes minor surgical corrections are beneficial in improving denture support. These include the following:

- frenectomy;
- excision of fibrous ridge/bands;
- reduction of enlarged tuberosities;
- contouring the bone (e.g. removal of exostoses or tori);
- removal of retained roots.

However, when severe bone resorption has taken place, other procedures may include:

- buccal vestibuloplasty;
- deepening of the floor of the mouth;
- augmentation of the bone;
- dental implants (see below);
- mental nerve repositioning;
- orthognathic surgery, occasionally used to correct gross jaw disproportion, enabling better control of the dentures.

Vestibuloplasty involves deepening the surrounding sulcus. Techniques include the use of mucosal flaps, or harvesting split-thickness mucosal or skin grafts.

Augmentation of the bone involves building up the deficient areas using autogenous bone or a synthetic material, such as hydroxyapatite. This is placed under the mucosa, where it hopefully integrates with the normal underlying bone to increase the height of the jaw. Augmentation may be used by itself or be required prior to the placement of implants.

Mental nerve repositioning may be required in grossly atrophic mandibles where the exit of the nerve from the bone has become superficial and compressed by the denture. Simply trimming back the denture often solves the problem, but in some cases the nerve is so superficial that this does not work. In such cases by using microsurgical techniques the nerve can be carefully dissected from its bony tunnel and repositioned away from the denture flange.

Osseo-integrated implants

The development of osseo-integrated implants has revolutionized the prosthetic rehabilitation of both totally and partially edentulous patients. Many patients who have undergone extensive treatment for oral cancer (see

Chapter 12) find it impossible to wear a 'suction' denture following surgery. However, by inserting implants into the residual mandible or into the reconstructed bone, construction of a retentive 'implant-borne' denture or bridge may be possible. Implant technology has enabled considerable improvements in functional rehabilitation with preservation of appearance. Psychological studies have also shown an inverse relationship between the ability to chew and depression. The need to provide a functioning prosthesis as early as possible after surgery is particularly important.

Denture rehabilitation should be considered *in the pre-operative assessment*, as this may affect the choice of reconstructive technique used. For instance, access to the mouth may be compromised following surgery (which restricts space for the denture), and by limitations in movements of the tongue, lip or mandible. Severe restrictions may also prevent effective oral hygiene. Rehabilitation should therefore not be reduced to an afterthought when inadequate reconstruction prevents implants from being used satisfactorily. Close co-operation between the surgeon, prosthedontist and maxillofacial technician is essential, as they are all dependent on each other for the planning and outcome of treatment. The patient needs to be sufficiently fit and motivated to undergo a prolonged course of treatment lasting up to 6–12 months following surgery. It is particularly important to exclude patients with psychiatric or specific medical disorders (e.g. depression or chronic alcoholism) who are likely to have problems with motivation and oral health.

In essence the technique involves the insertion into bone of implants or 'fixtures', as either a single or two-stage procedure, which become chemically bonded or 'osseo-integrated'. Osseo-integration is the direct and functional union of the bone with the implant surface under functional conditions such that osteoblasts can be seen on electron micrographs to be growing on the surface. In addition, a tight soft tissue attachment between the gums and the implant is essential. The fixtures form the foundations by which prostheses can be supported and retained (Fig. 16.1). Today implants are widely used for both intra-oral and extra-oral reconstruction. Many systems exist (screws, pins, transmandibular 'staples'), but most consist of cylindrical or screw-shaped titanium structures, sometimes coated with hydroxyapatite. Titanium is most commonly used, as it is extremely inert in the body, although gold and 'bioceramics' are occasionally used as alternatives.

Intra-oral implants

Intra-oral implants have many uses, ranging from replacement of a single tooth to whole-mouth rehabilitation (Fig. 16.2). The fixtures are placed in the bone following precise surgical preparation of a site that accurately fits the implant. Where multiple implants are to be used, great care is required to place them all parallel to each other. This is essential for further denture construction. Following placement, most implants are then buried beneath the mucosa during the period of osseo-integration in order to reduce the likelihood of infection. During osseo-integration the implants must be free of stress

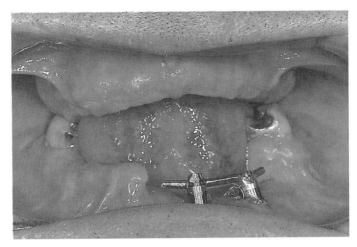

Figure 16.1   Osseo-integrated implant. The suprastructure attached to the implant provides the foundation supporting a partial denture.

as they must not undergo movement. The aim is to achieve direct contact between healthy vital bone and the surface of the implant. Post-operatively the maintenance of a high standard of oral hygiene and avoidance of smoking are essential.

Articulated 'study models' of both jaws are prepared on which a diagnostic 'wax-up' or trial prosthesis is constructed. From this the prosthodontist can consider how the implant fixtures relate to the dental arch. Following osseo-integration (about 3 months) the fixture is uncovered and a 'super-structure' is made which attaches to it. These include crowns, bridges and bar-retained dentures.

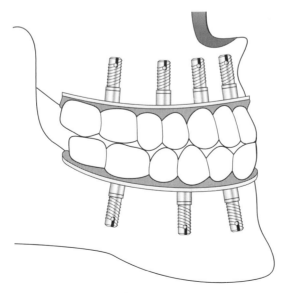

Figure 16.2   Implant-borne dentures.

Success depends on the following factors:

- the quality of the supporting bone;
- the surrounding mucosa;
- biocompatibility;
- biomechanical conditions post-operatively;
- continuous patient co-operation and excellent oral hygiene.

There must be sufficient bone (in terms of both height and width) to enable placement of the implants without damaging adjacent structures (the inferior alveolar nerve, maxillary sinus, floor of nose and adjacent teeth). Where not enough bone is present in the mandible, ridge augmentation as described previously may be necessary. In the maxilla, bone augmentation may require a Le Fort I osteotomy or a 'sinus lift', in which autogenous bone is placed beneath the lining of the maxillary sinus. Iliac crest, tibial and chin bone are all suitable donor sites. Bone 2 years after irradiation is generally considered to be suitable for implantation. Studies have shown a significant improvement in the survival of implants in irradiated bone with the use of hyperbaric oxygen therapy before and immediately following placement.

The site and inclination of the implants must be such as to support forces of mastication and enable the construction of an aesthetic prosthesis. In some cases additional surgical procedures such as vestibuloplasty, bone augmentation and osteotomy may be required. 'Functional loading' of the implants results in forces being directed towards the jaw, which helps to preserve the residual bone.

The thickness and mobility of the overlying soft tissues is also important. Ideally, a tightly bound mucoperiosteum should be present, whereas full-thickness skin grafts or thick mobile mucosa predispose towards inflammation and infection.

Complications of implants

These include the following:

- pain;
- peri-implantitis and infection;
- numbness;
- mandibular fracture;
- bone resorption;
- damage to adjacent teeth;
- mobile implant/loss of implant;
- osteoradionecrosis.

Extra-oral (facial) implants

Implants can also be used in the treatment of facial disfigurement using prostheses. The excellent quality and likeness of 'false' noses, ears and eyes to the real thing now means that replacement of these lost tissues can be accomplished without the need for multiple reconstructive procedures, which often give inferior results. Surgery itself is also much simpler and can often be carried out under local anaesthesia. 'Percutaneous' implants are also used for the retention of temporal bone-anchored hearing aids.

As a result of eliminating the need for adhesives, skin reactions are now uncommon. Patients no longer need to wear spectacle frames for orbital prostheses. Implants can now be placed in the orbit, mastoid, nasal and other regions of the face. Success rates are generally in excess of 95 per cent, although following irradiation this figure may be lower. Different systems are used as the bone is generally thinner. However, as with intra-oral implants where bone support is inadequate, augmentation or reconstruction can be carried out using iliac crest, calverial bone or microvascular free-tissue transfer (free flaps).

The principles are similar to those of intra-oral implants. The fixtures are inserted into the bone via small skin incisions, which are then closed immediately to form a watertight seal. Sites at risk during implant insertion include the dura, the sigmoid venous sinus, the frontal, ethmoid and maxillary air sinuses and the ear canal. After a minimum period of 3 months, they are exposed and subcutaneous tissue is removed in order to minimize skin mobility. Occasionally skin grafts may be required. 'Couplings' are placed and the skin incision is closed around the penetrating metal. Dressings after surgery are important and need to be repeated for several weeks before construction of the prosthesis or fitting of the hearing aid can begin. After tissue swelling has settled, impressions are taken for construction of the definitive prosthesis. The prosthesis must not be harmful to the skin, and for this reason most prostheses are made from medical-grade silicones. Unfortunately, the materials currently available are not very durable (silicones are easily damaged) and they do not retain their colour well. Replacement of prostheses after about 2 years is therefore necessary.

Success rates with orbital and nasal implants are lower, possibly due to the different quality of the bone in these sites. Usually more implants are placed than are actually required, so that some can be kept in reserve.

17 Maxillofacial surgery in children

Sally Wharnsby and Michael Perry

General points
Cleft lip and palate
Problems associated with cleft lip and palate
Management of cleft lip and palate
Paediatric craniofacial deformity
Trauma and emergency admissions
Useful addresses

Children undergoing maxillofacial surgery need to be admitted to specialist units that can meet their necessary surgical, psychological and developmental needs. The most common reasons for admission of children to maxillofacial units are for elective surgery and following accidents.

The purpose of this chapter is therefore to outline the range and scope of maxillofacial surgery within the paediatric setting, and to provide information on children who experience either planned hospital admissions for surgery or those who are admitted as an emergency following injury.

General points

Pre-operative assessment and care

By the age of 7 years, a large number of children in the UK will have experienced their first hospital admission. Many of these will have been as a day case, promoting the paediatric philosophy of reducing hospital admissions and in-patient stay. Children should not be admitted to hospital unless it is necessary, and their length of stay should be as short as possible. All children receiving hospital care require preparation for their admission so that they will know what to expect in terms of the environment and facilities, medical procedures and nursing staff. Pre-admission programmes can enable both the child and their family to gain insight into the effect of admission, allowing the child to adjust more easily to the idea of hospital. Preparation and information have been shown to reduce anxieties associated with hospital admission, and children can be sent pre-admission paediatric booklets prior to their surgery. This rationale is based on the principle that fear of the known is less traumatic than fear of the unknown.

Every child should receive attention that is individually tailored to their needs and those of their family. The health-care needs of children differ considerably from those of adults. The specific needs of children in hospital are best addressed if specialist staff provide the care, and the paediatric nurse must base this on the needs of the whole family. Facilities for children must be separate from those for adults because of the wide differences in their needs. They should also be appropriate for that age group.

A large number of children have minor operations to the mouth, and in most circumstances these are carried out on a day-case basis under a short general anaesthetic. Common dento-alveolar procedures include:

- treatments that will facilitate orthodontics (e.g. removal of misplaced or impacted teeth);
- extractions for dental caries;
- disorders affecting the oral mucosa;
- oral cysts.

Ideally children admitted for day-case treatment should be placed at the beginning of the list as they require only a short period of treatment and can then be discharged as soon as they have recovered. This also ensures that children are fasted appropriately. Normal practice is such that fasting 4 h for light diet and milk feeds and clear fluids such as squash 2 h pre-operatively will usually ensure an empty stomach in children.

All children should be allocated a named nurse to provide orientation to the ward and to carry out the admission process. Children should be involved in this process and, if appropriate, should be involved in the decision-making process concerning their stay in hospital. All aspects of treatment must be explained to both the child and their family, including both pre- and post-operative care, focusing on the sensory aspects of the experience and any concerns/anxieties. The use of a topical local anaesthetic cream should be common practice for all children undergoing a general anaesthetic, and it should be applied to the back of the child's hands 1–2 h prior to anaesthetic induction. This has revolutionized the comfort of the child during cannulation in the anaesthetic room. All parents should be given the choice of escorting their child to the anaesthetic room and staying until the child is asleep, as most children depend on their parents for emotional support and help in coping with anxiety. The next time the parents will see their child will be in the recovery unit, and they should be prepared with regard to their child's likely appearance and behaviour. Any minor surgery to the mouth will result in a small amount of oozing from the fresh operation sites; this is normal and should stop soon. Once recovered, the child will be nursed in the lateral position, allowing any blood to flow out of the mouth and not down the throat. Once awake, they should be encouraged to sit up slowly, in order to reduce the post-operative swelling.

Post-operative care

Children recover very quickly from short anaesthetics and soon require, as appropriate, something to drink and eat. They will probably only wish to take a soft diet for a few days, although there are no particular dietary restrictions. Encouraging the child to drink clear fluids following a meal will aid the commencement of oral hygiene. Keeping the child's mouth clean is very important. Stiffness of the jaw may restrict mouth-opening for a while, but the child should be encouraged to continue normal tooth-cleaning from the first day after surgery. Any vigorous mouth cleaning should be avoided for the first 24 h in order to leave the surgical site undisturbed.

All children should be given appropriate analgesia peri- and post-operatively, and it is essential for the nursing staff to observe and assess verbal and non-verbal signs of pain. Minor oral surgery to the mouth causes pain and discomfort, and the administration of medication to children is one of the nurse's most important responsibilities. Safety and competence are major issues in terms of delivering the correct dose in the least traumatic manner. Initially post-operatively the child's pain should be *anticipated* and an appropriate analgesic given, rather than having to ease the pain once it has developed. *Regular* analgesia should then be taken as necessary, not exceeding the recommended dose. The discomfort may be greater 1 or 2 days after the operation, after which time it should steadily decrease.

Facial swelling following minor surgery to the mouth varies, and the child and their family should be warned that it normally peaks on the second or third post-operative day. This swelling may take several days to resolve, and can be further reduced by nursing the child in an upright position.

Once the child has recovered fully from both the surgery and the anaesthetic, they will be discharged. Their recovery involves the toleration of both fluid and solid diet, the passing of urine after surgery and the absence of any complications. The discharge instructions must be explicit so that the parents have clear information on when to contact the hospital for help and advice should there be a change in their child's condition. Complications include gross swelling, pyrexia and continued bleeding. The parents should be given the following simple steps to follow should obvious bleeding occur.

- Soak a clean handkerchief or gauze swab in hot water, squeeze it as dry as possible and roll one end into a small ball.
- Rinse the child's mouth and place the pack directly over the bleeding site.
- Encourage the child to bite or press on the pack for at least 15–20 min while resting quietly.
- Repeat as necessary.

The parents should be advised to stay calm and to contact the hospital should they require urgent assistance.

Most children who undergo minor surgery to the mouth experience an uneventful surgical procedure with a straightforward recovery and no further need for surgical intervention. Sutures are normally resorbable, and any follow-up can usually be by their own family dentist.

Children who require treatment for other specific conditions will be treated as in-patients. The same paediatric ethos will apply whether the admission is for 1 day or for longer. Children should always be nursed separately to adults, in a relaxed and child-friendly environment. They have the right to be nursed by skilled and appropriately trained nurses, to have a parent residing with them during their hospital stay, and to be protected from unnecessary medical treatment. All care must be given in the best interests of the child, and an important element of care is parental presence and participation. The parents should be involved and informed throughout their child's hospital admission, and 'family-centred care' is extremely important.

Cleft lip and palate

Clefts of the lip and/or palate are one of the most common malformations in the craniofacial region. The incidence of cleft lip and palate is about 1.25 per 1000 live births in the UK and Ireland (around 1000 new cases per year). However, it does vary in different parts of the world (e.g. approximately 2 per 1000 live births in Norway) and also according to the type of cleft, the sex of the child and their racial group. Clefts appear to develop as a result of a mixture of genetic and environmental factors. Some types have a family history, implying a genetic predisposition, whereas others seem to be related more to environmental factors. Phenytoin (e.g. taken in pregnancy) has been shown to increase the incidence of cleft lip and palate.

Embryology

Facial development is a complex process which is still not fully understood. Between 7 and 8 weeks *in utero*, mesodermal migration results in the fusion of various 'facial processes' to form the upper lip. Cleft lip results from a failure of growth and fusion of these processes. In most cases tissues are not actually missing but merely underdeveloped and misplaced.

Most of the hard palate and the soft palate is formed from 'palatal shelves' which fuse in the mid-line during the first 6 weeks of intrauterine life. Normally, fusion is initially prevented by a relatively large tongue, but as the oral cavity enlarges and the neck extends, this enables the palatal shelves to meet and fuse in the mid-line together with the 'primary' palate anteriorly and the nasal septum above. Failure of this fusion leads to clefting of the 'secondary' palate. In some cases inadequate mesodermal fusion can give rise to a 'submucous' cleft in which the mucosal lining is intact but there is no bone or muscle in between.

As a result of the abnormal function of the muscles of the soft palate and upper lip, secondary deformities of the underlying facial skeleton occur.

Dental anomalies

In addition to the cleft there may also be an increased incidence of hypodontia (missing teeth) and supernumerary teeth (extra teeth), especially in the region of the cleft. The teeth themselves may also be malformed and their eruption delayed.

Classification

'Cleft lip and palate' covers a wide group of patients, each of which requires different management, depending on the amount of clefting present and the structures involved. In essence the deformity involves three muscle 'sphincters' and associated skin, mucosa, cartilage and bone. The three sphincters are the oral sphincter, the velopharyngeal sphincter and the nasal sphincter. Thus severe clefting of the lip and palate involves the disruption of:

- the oral sphincter (orbicularis oris);
- the velopharyngeal sphincter (levator veli palatini, tenser veli palatini, palato pharyngeas, palato glossus, muscularis uvulae and superior pharyngeal constrictor);
- the nasal sphincter (orbicularis oris and levator labiae superioris alaqui nasi).

Many classifications exist, but the best approach is probably to describe the cleft. Kurnerhan and Stark developed a classification based on the embryology of the deformity. The incisive foramen (just behind the upper central incisor teeth on the hard palate) is regarded as the demarcation between 'primary' and 'secondary' palates (see Box 17.1).

BOX 17.1 Classification of cleft lip and palate

- Clefts of the primary palate. 'Primary' refers to a cleft of the lip and/or palate anterior to the incisive foramen
- Clefts of the secondary palate. 'Secondary' refers to a cleft of the palate posterior to the foramen
- Clefts of the primary and secondary palate

Each of these may be 'complete' or 'incomplete', unilateral or bilateral. A bilateral complete cleft lip and palate is characterized by forward displacement of the premaxilla.

Cleft lip ranges from simple notching of the lip to a complete cleft, involving the lip, floor and base of the nose (Fig. 17.1), and it may be associated with a cleft of the primary palate (alveolus/premaxilla). It may also be associated with clefts of the secondary palate (hard and soft palate), which may be unilateral or bilateral.

Cleft palate may occur in isolation or it may be associated with a cleft lip. In its least affected form, a cleft palate involves a cleft of the muscles alone, with an intact mucosal lining and a bifid uvular – the submucous cleft. Alternatively, it may involve the posterior two-thirds of the hard palate, and all of the soft palate.

Facial growth

Adults with *unrepaired* clefts show very little difference in facial growth compared to the normal population. However, following repair, patients often develop a characteristic mid-facial retrusion. This is secondary to scarring *as a result of surgery*, which restricts the normal forward growth of the maxilla. The mandible is relatively unaffected, leading to the mistaken impression that it is oversized. The type of surgery, timing and technique are therefore important factors influencing the severity of growth disturbances.

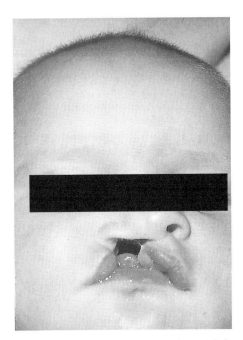

Figure 17.1 Complete unilateral cleft lip with associated nasal deformity.

Problems associated with cleft lip and palate

Disruption of the three sphincters causes functional problems and cosmetic disfigurement.

BOX 17.2 Functional and cosmetic impairment

Feeding. Inability to suck. Usually in cleft palate, but may occur with cleft lip.

Nasal regurgitation. This is caused by the communication between the mouth and nasal cavity. Coughing and chest infections may develop during feeding.

Hearing. In cleft palate the muscles of the Eustachian tube are affected, resulting in poor drainage of fluid in the middle ear. If left untreated, deafness can result.

Speech problems. These are related to:
- palatal defects;
- poor hearing;
- dentoalveolar defects;
- velopharyngeal incompetence (VPI) (see below).

Dentition. The upper lateral incisors and the canines are usually abnormally positioned, and there may be supernumerary teeth. The importance of dental hygiene must be stressed, because good orthodontics is impossible without it.

Respiratory. Displacement of the nasal septum may contribute to chronic sinusitis and chest infections.

Appearance. There may be:
- unsightly cleft lip;
- when unilateral, asymmetry of the nasal tip, alar dome and alar base. The nasal septum is also displaced;
- in bilateral clefts there is a short columella and splayed nasal tip;
- retruded mid-face and misalignment of the dental arches as the patient grows older.

Management of cleft lip and palate

The Royal College of Surgeons Steering Group on Cleft Lip and Palate has recommended minimum standards of care for these patients. These include the following.

- A team approach, including specialized counselling, specialized nursing, maxillofacial surgery, plastic surgery, orthodontics, dental care, speech and language therapy, otology/audiology, clinical genetics and developmental paediatrics is essential.
- Co-ordination of the team is needed from a single regional centre where registration of cases, record-keeping, treatment planning and multidisciplinary audit are undertaken. There should be regular courses for

non-team members (e.g. health visitors, midwives, paediatricians and speech and language therapists).

- Neo-natal counselling – an experienced professional should assess the child on the first day of life and provide the parents with reassurance and information on the future programme of management.
- Neo-natal nursing – a nurse specialist in the team should give early instructions to the mother on feeding and nursing. Separation of the mother and child should be kept to an absolute minimum.
- Surgery – this should be performed only by experienced surgeons with extended training in cleft lip and palate and frequent involvement in this work.
- Surgery should conform to well-tried protocols unless alternative procedures are introduced as part of an ethically approved surgical trial. Surgical records should include photographs and detailed anatomical descriptions of the pre-operative cleft, preferably augmented by dento-facial casts obtained at the time of primary surgery.
- Orthodontic treatment should be performed only by experienced orthodontists with extended cleft lip and palate training.
- Dental health education should be commenced by a named member of the team. Children with repaired clefts should have priority access to a consultant in paediatric dentistry where necessary.
- A specialist speech and language therapist should carry out early counselling and diagnostic assessment, and provide the necessary therapy either directly or through liaison with a local therapist.
- Otology audiology assessment.
- Clinical genetics.
- Psychological counselling (see below).
- Paediatric developmental medicine.
- Audit and research – the cleft lip and palate team should be subject to regular audit. The team should participate in multicentre audits and in national and international research.
- A parent support group should be available.

A thorough understanding of facial growth is essential if cleft lip and palate is to be treated successfully. Patients often require frequent admissions for surgical procedures throughout their school years and into adulthood, and familiarity with the team is helpful in developing a rapport.

Antenatal diagnosis

By week 14 of gestation, the facial contour is virtually complete, so detection of cleft lip may be possible as early as the end of the first trimester. The evidence suggests that cleft lip is detectable by transvaginal sonography, but this is not a standard scan for detection of fetal malformations. The usual transabdominal sonographic examinations have not been successful in detecting clefts. The advantages of prenatal diagnosis include the opportunity to prepare the child's parents in advance with regard to the presence of a cleft lip, enabling counselling and the opportunity for them to meet parents of other cleft-lip children. In some countries it also offers the possibility of offering termination at an early stage.

Immediate and early management

Parents are naturally very distressed when they find that their child has a cleft, and they may undergo denial or even rejection of the infant. Careful counselling at an early stage is necessary. Every child should ideally be seen by the surgical team within days of birth. The team will be multidisciplinary, including an experienced specialist nurse with the skills and knowledge to help the parents to come to terms with their child's abnormality. During this initial visit the surgeon and specialist nurse share their knowledge with the parents and teach the family members the appropriate skills they will require to meet their child's needs effectively. This counselling support will cover body image, enabling the parents to discuss their feelings about their child's condition. The speech and language therapist can also give advice on what feeding problems are to be expected, and their management.

Many parents find it useful to meet children with similar clefts (that have been repaired) and their parents. During the initial assessment the family should be introduced to local support groups such as the Cleft Lip And Palate Association (CLAPA), which can be contacted for information and support, feeding equipment and the sharing of experiences. The association is run by both parents and professionals, who share their unique experience and knowledge with the parents of newly born children. If the specialist nurse service is unavailable to your particular obstetric unit, NHS Trust or district general hospital, then telephone your nearest specialist unit or CLAPA for advice. This service should exist as part of the team supporting these families.

Screening for other congenital deformities is essential, the treatment of which may take precedence.

Feeding may be a problem, and infants with cleft palate may experience nasal regurgitation if there is any oronasal communication. Feeding methods should be assessed and discussed and the wishes of the parents taken into consideration. If the mother wants to breastfeed and the baby has the ability to suck, this should be encouraged. If the baby is unable to suck, a range of bottles and teats specially designed for babies with clefts can be used. The specialist nurse will decide which type is best for the baby, and will support the parents throughout the feeding regime. Each baby requires time to establish a feeding pattern, and a specialist nurse will support the parents and baby as they do so.

In cleft palate, inadequate drainage of the Eustachian tubes predisposes the child to middle-ear infections. Eustachian tubes normally open through the action of the palatal musculature, which in large clefts can be abnormal. Hearing loss must be assessed by regular examination, tympanometry and audiometry. The combination of poor hearing and palatal incompetence, if left untreated, will interfere with speech development and educational progress. Myringotomies, middle-ear drainage and grommet insertion are often required.

Pre-surgical orthodontics

Pre-surgical orthodontics (pre-surgical orthopaedics) is recommended by some authorities, although its use is controversial. The aim is to improve the alignment of the upper gum pads and ultimately the upper dental arch, hopefully thereby facilitating surgery. Plates are fitted within the first few days in order to align the pads. These may also aid feeding by separating the mouth and nasal cavity. Pre-surgical orthodontics is claimed to be especially useful in bilateral cleft lip and palate where the premaxillary segment has rotated forwards and upwards. However, many centres have now abandoned pre-surgical orthopaedics, reserving it just for severe cases. At an early stage it is also important to make visual records and study models.

Principles of surgical management and nursing care

Surgery aims to restore normal anatomy and physiology in order to encourage normal facial development. This involves accurate reconstruction of the muscles of the lip and soft palate. The timing of surgery and the techniques used vary between centres. However, in all cases it is important to be realistic and not to create unreasonably high expectations.

BOX 17.3 A 'typical' protocol for cleft lip and palate

- Repair of lip at 6–24 weeks
- Repair of the palate at 6–12 months
- Pharyngoplasty – not always necessary
- Alveolar bone grafting at 9–11 years
- Secondary revisions of the lip and nose
- Facial osteotomies at 15+ years
- Final rhinoplasty at 16+ years

Although in other countries the repair of cleft lip and palate has been carried out *in utero*, this approach is currently regarded as experimental, controversial and not without risks. Early repair of the lip is essential for the development of an oral seal to facilitate feeding, and closing of the palate must be undertaken prior to speech training.

Primary surgery

Lip repair is usually undertaken at around 6–24 weeks, although the timing and technique depend on the normal practice of the surgeon and the general condition of the infant. Many different procedures have been described (e.g. Millard, Le Mesurier and Tennyson, or their modifications), all of which attempt to produce a functioning lip of adequate length that is not too tight. The evidence now suggests that, in cleft lip, the orbiculus oris muscle is abnormally inserted into the margins of the cleft. These fibres need to be realigned in order to obtain normal function (Delaire procedure).

Pre-operative care

All families should be offered a pre-admission visit to the ward during their out-patient appointment to meet the team of nurses who will care for them and their baby. During this visit the nursing staff can advise the parents against the use of dummies prior to the surgery. Dummies are also avoided post-operatively if possible, as the constant sucking motion applies tension to the lip. During this visit the parents can be shown photographs of previous babies before and after surgical correction, so that the anxious parents can be reassured of the excellent results that can be produced by modern surgery.

The baby is usually admitted on the day prior to surgery, and photographs of the cleft lip are taken. He or she will need to have blood taken for a full blood count according to the hospital protocol. Ideally, the blood profile must show a haemoglobin level above 10 g/dl for surgery to take place. The baby must also be in good health, with no recent coughs or colds, and be feeding and gaining weight appropriately.

The parents should be included in all aspects of their baby's pre-operative preparation, and are encouraged to be resident in the hospital. All procedures are explained to them and information given about what to expect during the hospital stay. The parents should be encouraged to share their fears and anxieties, especially with regard to coping with the stress of their baby being in hospital for an operation. During the pre-operative period, nursing staff can discuss aspects of parental participation, feeding methods, pain control and facial appearance, all of which will change post-operatively. The baby may have nasal sponges and stents *in situ* post-operatively to shape the nose, and some babies may need arm restraints. The parents should be informed of these procedures prior to seeing their baby post surgery.

A pre-operative last milk feed should be given around 4 h before surgery, or as requested by the anaesthetist. The parents may then escort their baby to the anaesthetic room if they wish.

Post-operative care

The recovery technique and positioning used for airway maintenance of cleft-lip babies immediately after surgery involves nursing them on their side with a head-down tilt. Oxygen is given until the baby's oxygen saturation remains stable. Pain control is vital, as is accurate pain assessment by the nursing staff. During surgery the surgeon will have infiltrated the lip with a local anaesthetic to ensure a pain-free recovery. However, if the baby requires further analgesia morphine can be given. Alert observation of vital signs will continue as frequently as necessary until they are stable. Pain is one of the earliest signs that the baby can express verbally and non-verbally following surgery, so pain relief is of vital importance to maintain their comfort. Prompt administration of pain-relieving medication will avoid the situation of a fretful crying baby who may find it difficult to re-establish feeding post-operatively. Analgesia should be given regularly until the baby becomes settled and is able to feed well. This must be explained to the parents so that they know the difference between a cry of pain and one of hunger.

The parents should be present as soon as their baby is maintaining his or her own airway to provide cuddles, security and comfort. An uncomfortable baby will cry, and this can increase the tension across the surgical site. Steristrips or similar support are usually placed across the upper lip to prevent this tension, and arm splints/elbow restraints may be necessary to prevent little hands from touching the lip, and to protect the surgical site. Early feeding is encouraged to keep the baby content and comfortable, and the parents should be supported in participating in their baby's care as much as they feel able to. A contented baby has less chance of bleeding post-operatively causing further disruption to the lip. Intravenous fluids are maintained for hydration until oral feeding has been successfully re-established. The parents need to be supported through the period of re-introduction of feeding, as their baby may not feed initially due to the strange 'feel' of the surgical site. The baby's first feed can be glucose water, half- or full-strength feed, depending on the surgeon's preference. The use of bottle teats as a form of comfort should be avoided, and they should be removed from the baby's mouth on completion of the feed, to prevent continuous tension on the lip.

The nursing staff must support the parents when they see their baby for the first time. If the cleft lip is surgically repaired from 3–4 months onwards, the parents may experience a sense of loss for the 'pre-repair' baby. They should be encouraged to discuss their feelings about the child's altered body image and be supported through this grieving process.

Following an uneventful recovery the baby can be transferred back to the paediatric ward. The post-operative care is directed towards supporting the parents, pain relief, feeding requirements, splintage and wound care. The parents need to be supported through all aspects of the post-operative period, with explanations of all treatment given and reassurance given whenever necessary.

Post-operatively, a normal feeding regime should be encouraged, but the baby will need to get used to their newly shaped lip. Soft or specially designed teats (e.g. Habermann teat) can be used to aid feeding. The baby may have difficulty in breathing and feeding if nasal stents and sponges are *in situ*, depending on the surgeon's preference. A fluid-balance sheet will be maintained to ensure adequate intake. If the baby tires while feeding, smaller but more frequent amounts of feed will be necessary.

The lip repair must be protected over the next few weeks and, as well as wearing arm splints, the baby should not be positioned in any way that will allow the lip area to come into contact with bed clothing when they are asleep or an adult's body when they are being carried. The baby must not be carried or winded over the shoulder, as contact can cause damage to the lip. Arm splints, if worn, are required until the surgical site has healed, and their use can normally be discontinued on removal of the sutures 4–5 days post-operatively. The parents should be advised to remove the splints periodically to allow their baby a full range of movement and relief from the restrictions.

The surgical site and lip sutures must be kept clean, and this is important for optimum healing. A normal saline solution is used to cleanse the area gently and carefully, ensuring that the suture line is free of serous leakage, crust formation and milk-feed deposits. The surgical site should be inspected and cleaned after each feed. Any inflammation or changes in lip appearance must be reported to the surgeon immediately, as this could affect the final aesthetic result. Antibiotics may be prescribed for the baby if the surgical site indicates this. Monitoring of vital signs (e.g. temperature) will alert nursing and medical staff to the possibility of wound infection. The parents can encourage their baby to drink a clear fluid following each feed in order to keep the oral area clean. Steristrips are re-applied as necessary to maintain support and protection of the lip.

Only when the parents are happy with their baby's condition will discharge planning begin. The parents should be given the option of staying in hospital until suture removal if they feel that they could not cope at home. The following explicit discharge information must be given.

- Keep the suture line clean with cotton buds and cooled boiled water.
- Continue feeding as normal.
- Give analgesia as required.
- Suture removal will be on ....
- Splints can be worn if you wish.
- The out-patient appointment will be on ....
- Please discourage your baby from sucking a dummy, especially if a palate repair is to be carried out later.
- Often the scar shortens and pulls the lip up a few weeks after repair.
- This phase will pass and the lip will lengthen again in time.

It is good practice for the staff to telephone the family soon after their discharge (1–2 days) in order to check that all is well.

PALATE REPAIR

In the normal soft palate the muscles form a sling which lifts the palate during speech and swallowing. However, in cleft palate these muscles run parallel to each other, inserting into the posterior edge of the hard palate. Repair is therefore directed towards realignment of these muscles. The aim is to produce a functional, long, mobile palate by reconstructing the muscle and mucosa. Cleft palate involves no cosmetic disfigurement, but poor repair can result in poor speech development and chronic hearing problems. Well-known techniques include those of Delaire and Von Langenbeck.

Since clefts vary considerably, the timing of repair also varies depending on the surgeon's preference. The arguments for closing the palate by 18 months are to enable normal function before speech is established, and to reduce nasal regurgitation. However, the disadvantage of early repair is interference with mid-face growth. Some authorities argue in favour of delaying hard palate repair until 5 years or more after earlier repair of the soft palate. However, this view is controversial.

Nursing care for the cleft-palate repair has similarities to that for the cleft-lip repair, although the management of cleft palate can be more difficult. The family should have received support and guidance from members of the multidisciplinary team within days of their baby's birth. Babies with a cleft palate (depending on the extent) may require extra help and support with feeding, due to the inability to form a vacuum inside their mouth and suck. Some mothers, if given suitable encouragement, are able to breastfeed (depending on the severity of the cleft). The specialist cleft lip/palate nurse will assess and advise on a suitable feeding plan for each individual baby, supplying the different types of bottles and teats required. The type of feeding equipment and rate of feeding must be individualized for each baby. The surgeon may consider the use of a dental feeding plate to assist the baby. An orthodontist will provide this, although it is not required in the majority of cases. Some babies may have been diagnosed as having a condition called Pierre Robin syndrome, which consists of a small lower jaw (micrognathia), a cleft palate and glossoptosis, which allows the normal-sized tongue to fall back and block the child's airway, especially during feeding. A dental feeding plate can be used in this situation to fill the cleft and prevent the tongue from falling into the nasopharynx. Nasogastric-tube feeding may also be used in babies with this condition, to prevent cyanotic and choking episodes during feeding. All cleft-palate babies have the additional increased risk of aspiration while feeding, and the parents will be taught the specific techniques to use to make feeding time safe and enjoyable.

Pre-operative care

The pre-operative 'work-up' for the cleft-palate baby should be the same as that for babies with a cleft-lip repair, i.e. photographs, blood test, assessment by medical and anaesthetic teams, and explanations, support and guidance from the nursing team. In addition, the child may be seen by an ear, nose and throat surgeon, who will examine the ears and insert grommets, if indicated, while the child is having the palatal repair. Depending on local protocol, the child may also commence a course of prophylactic antibiotics in view of the surgical site, as the mouth and suture line are constantly being contaminated.

The parents need to be advised on the feeding method required prior to the surgical repair. Ideally the baby should be feeding from a small soft teat, spoon bottle or feeding cup/beaker. This is to prevent contact with the palate following surgical repair, and the parents should be advised to practise these feeding methods prior to surgery. The use of dummies and/or long, hard bottle teats is discouraged post-operatively, as it is thought that they may have an effect on the healing of the surgical site, due to their position in the mouth and the constant pressure on the suture line.

The nursing staff need to prepare the parents concerning what to expect post-operatively, and also need to encourage their participation in every aspect of their child's treatment and care.

Post-operative care

The child should be positioned for airway maintenance until he or she is conscious from the anaesthetic. Effective analgesia (e.g. morphine) should be given immediately to prevent the child from having a painful recovery. Intravenous fluid should be maintained at around 4 ml/kg per hour until the child is taking adequate oral fluids. Initially the child may have difficulty in re-establishing a breathing pattern, with the closure of the palatal defect, and the child's adopted pattern of breathing will need to be altered to breathing through the nose. The child's respiratory effort must be observed, but seldom needs anything other than a change in position. Occasionally they may have a tongue suture *in situ*, which can be used to prevent airway obstruction. This is common in children with Pierre Robin syndrome, and is usually removed 24 h after surgery.

Palatal blood loss must be monitored and reported to the surgeon if it does not cease. Oral suctioning should be avoided if possible, as this can disrupt the newly repaired palate. In most cases palatal bleeding will settle and the child should be prevented from crying by giving adequate analgesia, having plenty of cuddles from its parents and being fed when hungry. The child should be prevented from crying, as this will increase the tension on the suture line.

Feeding should be re-established as soon as the child can tolerate it, and clear fluids should be given following each milk feed in order to cleanse the mouth of any deposits, so keeping the suture line clean. Depending on the age of the child at repair, solids can be re-introduced at this stage so long as a clear fluid drink is given afterwards. The palate must also be kept clean following the administration of sticky oral medications such as analgesics and antibiotics.

Arm splints can also be used to keep the child's hands away from his or her mouth, in order to prevent injury to the suture line. Care must be taken when feeding the child solids. The diet must be soft and parents should take care when introducing eating utensils into the mouth. If teeth are present, the parents must be encouraged to maintain a high standard of oral hygiene, but should be advised to exercise caution around the surgical repair.

The child's comfort and feeding status will be reviewed regularly by the surgeon, and discharge planning will begin when the child is feeding well, apyrexial and pain-free. If there are no complications and the parents are not concerned, the child can be discharged from the second day following surgery. On the day of discharge the family will be seen by the speech therapist, and this liaison will begin the planned monitoring of the child's speech and language development. All aspects of post-operative care should be discussed with the parents and given as discharge advice to be adhered to until the follow-up appointment. Soft diet and oral hygiene are of the utmost importance. The family will later attend a combined joint clinic which recognizes the need for close collaboration with all the specialists involved in the child's care and further treatment.

BOX 17.4 Complications of primary surgery

- Lip dehiscence
- Palatal dehiscence is more common, especially if this becomes infected. Pre-operative nasal and throat swabs are therefore useful
- Oronasal fistulas – these require obturation or closure at a later stage using local palatal flaps or tongue flaps
- Secondary effects on facial growth (see section on secondary surgery)

Intermediate surgery

Alveolar bone grafting (ABG) involves using bone, often from the iliac crest or tibia, to close the bony defect in the alveolus. The bone stabilizes the upper arch, increases support for the base of the nose, aids the closure of oronasal fistulae and provides support for the adult canine tooth to erupt through. An intact upper arch also aids orthodontic treatment to close the space. Surgery is performed before the permanent canine erupts, and normally takes place when the child is around 9–10 years of age. Attempts have been made to close the alveolar defect early, at the time of the primary lip repair. However, the results obtained have generally been disappointing.

Pre-operative care

The child is admitted to hospital on the day before surgery to allow time to collect information that will enable the medical and nursing staff to plan his or her individualized care. The child and their parents should continue to be informed and participate in all decisions regarding care and treatment. Children need to be sure that although they are in an unfamiliar environment they are still in control of what happens to them. If they undergo pre-admission preparation they will usually know what to expect, and their stay in hospital should be as comfortable and enjoyable as possible.

During the collection of admission details, the nursing staff can begin to discuss the pre- and post-operative expectations with the child. If the child is prepared pre-operatively they will tend to comply post-operatively. They will be told that they will have two operation sites when they wake up from their anaesthetic, namely the mouth and the bone donor site (iliac crest or tibia). They should be told that the donor site will cause more discomfort than the mouth. The importance of strict oral hygiene will also be discussed. Pre-operative blood samples and X-rays will be taken as requested by the surgeon, and the child will be fasted appropriately.

Post-operative care

As soon as the child has regained consciousness and is maintaining their own airway, they should be nursed in an upright position in order to reduce any intra-oral swelling. The surgical site will be observed for bleeding and the child allowed to rest. Appropriate peri-operative analgesia will be given to ensure a pain-free post-operative period. If the iliac crest is used as the donor area, the child may have a long-acting local anaesthetic infusion (bupivacaine) to the site. This donor area can be more painful than the tibia, and will also affect the child's mobility in the initial post-operative period. The donor areas should be observed regularly, especially the iliac region, as this has the potential to bleed in the first 72 h following surgery.

Fluids can be taken as soon as they can be tolerated, continuing to a soft diet as the child wishes, and strict oral hygiene must be maintained. Vigorous mouthwashes and tooth-brushing are not recommended in the initial 24-h period, in order to prevent any dislodging of clot formation at the surgical site resulting in further bleeding. Due to the contamination of the mouth and surgical site, the child will be prescribed a course of antibiotic therapy and medicated mouthwashes to promote healing. Mouth care must be carried out after all dietary intake and following the administration of sticky medicines. Plastic eating utensils can be used initially, and the child should be discouraged from using straws for drinking, in order to prevent damage to the surgical site.

The child should be given regular appropriate analgesia to ensure a comfortable post-operative period, enabling them to eat and mobilize without any complications. If an infusion is used for an iliac donor, the nurse can assess the child's level of pain and increase or decrease the dose as required until the infusion is no longer needed. This will be effective when the child is up and fully mobile with no pain. Children tend to mobilize more readily and ably when the donor area used is the tibia, thus shortening their stay in hospital.

Children are encouraged to be mobile as soon as they feel able and comfortable.

Sutures to the mouth are usually resorbable and will disappear as healing takes place. Donor-area sutures will need to be removed 10–14 days after surgery and should not cause any problems.

The child and their parents should be educated in and prepared to carry out any ongoing care required following discharge, specifically oral hygiene. The child will normally decide when he or she feels fit for discharge and, so long as there are no obvious complications, this can be from the first day postoperatively. The maxillofacial surgeon usually reviews the child approximately 1 week after discharge to ensure that the surgical site is healing, and then refers them back to the care of the orthodontist for further sequential orthodontic treatment.

PHARYNGOPLASTY

Following repair of the soft palate, attempts at speech must be monitored closely and the speech and language therapist is essential here. Scarring in the palate can lead to poor function and velopharyngeal incompetence (VPI), characterized by failure of the soft palate (velum) and pharyngeal walls to meet properly during speech. Features of VPI are increased nasal resonance, inappropriate air escape, weak volume, articulatory problems and, eventually, hoarseness from straining. VPI is a clinical diagnosis, but assessment is important in planning therapy.

Speech assessment is essential for:

- diagnosis;
- management;
- assessing outcome;
- comparison of techniques/centres.

This includes the assessment of:

- nasal escape of air;
- quality of nasal resonance;
- articulation;
- voice (hoarseness);
- overall intelligibility.

Speech and velopharyngeal function can be visualized using nasendoscopy, cineradiography and videofluoroscopy (see Chapter 7). This requires a co-operative child, usually 4 years of age or over. Measurement of VP function includes techniques such as aninometry (nasal airflow during speech), the oral nasal acoustic ratio (TONAR) and pressure-flow studies.

Various operations are available for the management of VPI. These include:

- no treatment;
- speech therapy;

- biofeedback;
- palate surgery;
- prosthetic treatment;
- pharyngoplasty.

Surgical technique is important, as pharyngoplasty may be followed by too tight a closure, resulting in nasorespiratory obstruction, with snoring, inability to clear nasal secretions, and sleep apnoea.

Secondary surgery

During growth, surgery to reconstruct tissues has an effect on further development, due to scar formation. Good technique is essential in order to minimize the amount of scar tissue formed. Untreated cleft patients are seen to have relatively normal facial development. Surgery is therefore a major factor and delaying primary surgery until the patient is older reduces growth disturbance. However, this must be balanced against the poor speech and hearing as well as the psychological impact associated with the deformity. Most secondary procedures should be deferred until growth is nearly complete.

'Secondary' cleft deformity is therefore the residual deformity resulting from:

- the original embryological defect;
- primary surgery;
- subsequent growth.

BOX 17.5   Secondary surgical procedures

- Orthognathic surgery to correct skeletal malrelationships (e.g. maxillary osteotomy, bimaxillary osteotomy)
- Further bone grafting to unite the maxillary segments
- Closure of palatal fistulae
- Septorhinoplasty
- Revision of the nose or lip in order to improve the appearance. A perfectly symmetrical nose tip is one of the more difficult targets to achieve. Many surgical procedures are available

Dental management

Cleft-palate patients frequently have inadequate plaque control, partly because of the dental irregularities and partly because of self-neglect due to prolonged treatment. It is essential that from an early age the parents are informed of the need for good dental care and preventive measures. Where fluoride levels in water are low, fluoride supplements should be given early. The child must also have regular dental inspections.

Paediatric craniofacial deformity

Paediatric craniomaxillofacial surgery has now emerged as a subspecialty in its own right. It is concerned with the treatment of rare and complex congenital or acquired anomalies of the head, upper face and jaws. Many of these may be associated with malformations in other parts of the body, particularly the following:

- cardiac region;
- renal region;
- cleft lip and palate;
- skeletal areas (e.g. hands);
- others.

Surgery for craniofacial deformity began in the late 1960s. The principles of craniofacial surgery are to aim to correct the deformity totally in a limited number of operations. This has resulted in fewer major complications than previously. Since the majority of patients are children, often undergoing surgery when they are less than 2 years old, comprehensive paediatric facilities are essential, including access to an intensive-care unit (ICU) or high-dependency unit (HDU). Surgery is often major, may threaten the airway, and often involves relatively large amounts of blood loss.

Craniosynostosis and craniofacialsynostosis

These conditions occur when there is premature fusion of the sutures between the bones of the skull. Single or multiple sutures may fuse, with the result that growth is restricted in certain directions. This leads to characteristic alterations in the shape of the skull and face. Craniosynostosis occurs in up to 1 per 2000 live births. The aetiology is unknown, although 20 to 40 per cent of cases show an inherited pattern. Premature fusion may lead to two main problems:

- raised intracranial pressure (with or without hydrocephalis), although this is more common where multiple sutures are involved;
- deformity of the cranial and facial skeleton.

Corrective surgery may be necessary in order to reduce intracranial pressure or correct the appearance. Since 50 per cent of skull growth is achieved by 6 months of age, early surgery is often required. A team approach is essential, involving a neurosurgeon, oral and maxillofacial surgeon, plastic surgeon, anaesthetist, paediatrician, ophthalmologist, orthodontist, paedadontist, prosthodontist, maxillofacial technician, psychologist, audiologist, geneticist and social worker. Most cases are now managed in designated craniofacial centres.

BOX 17.6   Indications for surgical correction

- Raised intracranial pressure
- Proptosis requiring ocular protection
- Inadequate airway
- Grotesque appearance
- Dental occlusal problems

Timing depends on the severity of these indications. Surgery involves release of the sutures and allowing normal growth to take place. Early surgery is required to prevent blindness and mental retardation, and opinions differ with regard to the optimum age for surgery, but about 3 months is generally acceptable. Where the face is also involved (craniofacial synostoses), treatment involves early release of the skull sutures to allow normal brain development and later advancement of the mid-face. This is usually carried out at around 16–18 years when growth is complete. However, early Le Fort III advancement may be necessary in cases where there is a significant risk of blindness from proptosis or severe sleep apnoea.

Diagnosis

This is usually clinical, as radiographic changes may be late. Examination includes assessment of the skull, cranial base, orbits and eyes, mid-face and nose, mouth and palate, dentition and occlusion and the lower face. Associated anomalies should also be looked for. Plain skull radiographs (Fig. 17.2), lateral cephalograms and MRI and CT scans may all be of value. Genetic assessment and counselling of the parents are also necessary at an early stage.

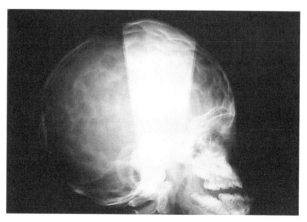

Figure 17.2   Craniofacial synostosis. Note the 'copper-beaten' appearance of the skull, suggesting raised intracranial pressure.

Pre-operative care

In the general assessment, motivational, psychological and emotional aspects must be taken into account, in addition to mental development. Many of these children suffer from airway difficulties secondary to narrowing of the nose and underdevelopment of the mid-face. Recurrent chest infections may occur and, if recent, will predispose to secondary infection, particularly after a prolonged anaesthetic. This should be assessed pre-operatively and any problems managed with physiotherapy, antibiotics, etc., to ensure the child is as fit as possible for surgery. Haemoglobin levels must be checked and the parents advised that blood transfusion is usually necessary. Emla cream should be applied and premedication given if necessary. Children are at a lower risk of developing DVTs than adults. Nevertheless, graduated compression stockings or inflating leggings are often used.

Surgical technique

Adequate exposure is important in the correction of craniofacial anomalies. This is usually via a coronal flap in which the skin incision extends across the top of the head, from ear to ear, well within the hairline. Dissection is then carried down over the front of the skull beneath the forehead, effectively a 'scalping' procedure. In this way good access to the skull, upper facial skeleton and orbits is possible while avoiding incisions on the face. Operative procedures include cranial expansion and orbital translocations.

Cranial expansion is performed where there is multiple suture fusion. Here the intracranial volume is increased by forward advancement of the forehead. In orbital translocations, abnormally positioned orbits are moved into a correct relationship with one another.

Surgery often involves exposure of the anterior cranial base, which is made possible by removing the frontal bones and retracting the brain and dura. The floor of the middle cranial fossa can also be accessed using this approach. Cuts can then be made in the bones so that they can be repositioned.

In the craniofacial synostoses, for instance, the forehead and supra-orbital margins are often moved forward. In addition, the orbits can be isolated and repositioned. Hypertelorism is caused by separation of the orbits, and may be associated with craniosynostosis, clefting defects and meningoencephaloceles. Minor deformity may be corrected without exposing the cranial cavity, but where there is gross deformity a transcranial procedure is necessary. Both orbits can then be repositioned medially, and the central nasal block of bone is removed.

The bones are fixed into their new positions by means of wires or miniplates. Any gaps that are created can be repaired using bone grafts taken from the cranium, ribs and iliac bone. Bone behaves differently in this region compared to other regions of the body. Large segments can be completely detached from their soft tissue attachments and yet survive and grow normally, so long as they do not become infected.

After completion of surgery, the scalp flap is repositioned on the skull and face. This approach means that there should be no scars on the face.

POST-OPERATIVE CARE

Careful supervision is essential, paying particular attention to fluid balance, heat loss and signs of intracranial complications. Admission to an ICU/HDU is therefore necessary in the immediate post-operative period, so that close monitoring is possible, which includes the following:

- airway;
- oxygenation;
- cardiovascular function;
- bleeding;
- signs of raised intracranial pressure;
- neurological signs;
- vision;
- urinary output;
- fluid balance;
- surgical drains.

In the early post-operative phase on return to the ward the patient still requires specialist nursing care and monitoring. Sutures and dressings are usually removed before the patient is discharged from hospital, but may be left longer. For patients living at a distance from the unit, arrangements are made locally for dressings and suture removal. Plain skull radiographs are obtained as soon as is practicable after surgery. Occasionally a further brief admission for monitoring of intracranial pressure may be required.

BOX 17.7 Complications (these are generally uncommon)

- Neurosurgical complications (CSF leakage, brain injury, meningitis, post-operative epilepsy)
- Ocular complications (blindness, nasolacrimal damage, ptosis, diplopia)
- Unrecognized blood loss, particularly in small children
- Airway problems
- Infection (wound, bone)
- Bitemporal hollowing
- Late problems due to relapse of the bone and soft tissue

Callous distraction

In some cases of craniofacial and hemifacial microsomia, callous distraction is a useful technique for enlarging the mandible during the growth phase. Following osteotomy of the bone, a miniature 'external fixator' is applied across the 'fracture' with a screw device, enabling the pins to be slowly separated, thereby pushing the bone ends apart (distraction). Small increments in distraction are applied daily, preventing the callus from uniting solidly until the desired length is reached. This technique is commonly used in limb-lengthening procedures in orthopaedic surgery. Up to a 25-mm increase in length has been recorded in the mandible. Facial asymmetries and mandibular retrognathia can be corrected in this way and improvement in the airways achieved. More recently developed distractors can now be placed intra-orally and are thus unobtrusive and avoid the major cheek scars that are associated with extra-oral appliances.

Free flaps

The availability of microvascular free tissue transfer, a procedure which was initially performed only in adults, has increased the options available for the management of complex craniofacial problems in infants and young children. Free tissue transfer provides vascularized tissue to close dead space, line internal surfaces and provide skin cover. Vascularized bone grafts are especially useful in the reconstruction of the paediatric mandible.

Cranial synostoses (skull only)

SINGLE SUTURE

Suture involved		Deformity
• Sagittal	→	scaphocephaly
• Unilateral coronal	→	plagiocephaly
• Metopic	→	trigonocephaly
• Lambdoid	→	posterior plagiocephaly

MULTIPLE SUTURES

• Bicoronal	→	brachycephaly
• Pan craniosynostosis		

Craniofacial synostosis – syndromes

- Crouzon's syndrome
- Acrocephalo-syndactyly syndromes:
    Apert's;
    Saethre–Chotzen;
    Pfeiffer's;
    Carpenter;
    others.

Many of these syndromes overlap.

Secondary craniosynostoses

These arise as a result of some other condition, such as hydrocephalus, microcephaly, rickets, hyperthyroidism, thalassaemia and drugs (e.g. diphenylhydantoin and retinoic acid).

Craniofacial clefting syndromes

These are different to cleft lip and palate and are numbered from 0 to 14, with the lower numbers representing facial clefts and the higher numbers representing their cranial extensions. Multiple and bilateral clefts can occur in the same patient.

Miscellaneous conditions

These include trauma, other craniofacial pathology and benign and malignant tumours.

Trauma and emergency admissions

A significant number of children are treated each year by maxillofacial units after sustaining traumatic injuries. An emergency admission to hospital can be one of the most stressful, frightening and anxious experiences for a child and their family. The injured child will be unprepared for what is about to happen and will need constant explanations. The parents should be allowed to stay with their child during all investigations and treatments, and they too will require support and information.

During an emergency admission children are often in pain, while at the same time being subjected to strange and unfamiliar surroundings which only increase their anxiety. Children need a calm, relaxed and unhurried admission process, whether it is planned or unplanned. Children are compliant if they are comfortable and pain-free, understand what is happening to them and have their parents with them. Most paediatric emergency admissions managed by maxillofacial units are not life-threatening, and time can be spent explaining the situation and preparing the child and their parents for their surgery and hospital stay. With emergency admissions there is a tendency to perform procedures and treatments quickly, and sometimes the child's needs can be overlooked. Any emergency admission is compounded by the need for surgery, and this may be the first time that the child has been admitted to hospital, let alone having to undergo a surgical procedure. All explanations that are given to the child must be age appropriate, allowing them to understand the care and treatment they will receive. Children need to participate in their care in order to maintain a sense of control and an understanding of all the events that take place.

Parental participation should be welcomed, as the child–parent relationship is unique and can help the child to cope with the special tests, procedures and surgery they may need to undergo. Parents know their child better than anyone else, and if they are supported and kept informed of their condition, this will benefit the child.

Paediatric maxillofacial injuries consist of damage to the soft tissue and facial skeleton as a result of falls, bicycle and road traffic accidents, contact and wounding, and sporting accidents.

Facial lacerations

Childhood accidents resulting in abrasions, scratches, cuts and bruises are generally regarded as the norm in a child's lifetime and do not normally necessitate surgical intervention. Depending on the size and depth of the injury, facial lacerations need to be assessed appropriately and treated accordingly. For most children this will involve a short general anaesthetic to repair the damage. Some cases can be treated under local anaesthetic, but this must only be undertaken with the full consent and co-operation of the child. Most children present with a facial wound that bleeds and appears to be quite deep. This can be extremely upsetting for both the child and their parents. Facial lacerations can bleed quite profusely and this adds to what is already a stressful and anxious situation. The initial treatment should be directed towards cessation of blood loss and cleaning of the wound. Only then can the surgeon assess the need for suturing. The wound should be toileted gently with a normal saline solution and a non-adhesive dressing applied. Analgesia should be given prior to this procedure if it is felt necessary by the child, parents and nursing staff. Depending on the cause of the accident, further examinations may be requested, such as an X-ray to detect any foreign bodies in the wound. The parents should always be asked whether the child was knocked out at the time of the accident, in order to ascertain other complications. If a head injury is suspected, then surgery should be delayed for 24 h and/or until neurological observations are stable. The child's tetanus status should always be established, especially when the wound appears dirty.

If there are no complications, the child should be taken to theatre as soon as possible. Children should only be fasted for the minimum period of time required for a safe general anaesthetic. The aim of surgery is to clean and debride the wound properly and to suture the laceration. The child and their parents should be warned of the possibility of post-operative bruising and swelling, and need to be reassured that this will settle quickly.

Post-operative care is directed towards ensuring a safe and uneventful recovery from the general anaesthetic, and care of the surgical site. Suture lines are normally left exposed to the air or supported by steristrips. Most surgeons prescribe a course of antibiotics for the child to take, especially if the wound was dirty, and this should be completed. The child's stay in hospital should be short, and they can be considered for discharge when they are fit. Post-operatively, the suture line will require daily cleaning with normal saline and the parents can be taught the correct technique to use at home. They can be shown and then supervised as they perform their child's wound care in hospital. Crust formation on the wound can prevent optimum healing, resulting in a larger scar. The parents should then be instructed on care of the wound at home and the child discharged. The sutures will be removed 4–5 days following surgery, and the parents should be instructed to telephone the ward if there are any problems. Depending on the number of sutures and the area of injury, the child could return to the ward or wound care clinic, or attend the family's general practitioner for removal of the sutures. If the wound has a large number of fine sutures and is in an awkward place, then an experienced nurse will need to remove them. Suture removal, especially on the face, should not be hurried and must only be attempted when the child is calm. Some children may require a light oral sedative prior to suture removal, as it is very important that the child lies still when this procedure is being carried out. Any sudden movement by the child can cause the suture to be pulled, causing unnecessary damage to the healing suture line. Great care must be taken to ensure integrity of the suture line. Occasionally it may be necessary to remove alternate sutures if there is uncertainty about the healing process. Following removal the repaired laceration can be supported with steristrips.

The parents should be advised to keep the steristrips in place until they fall off, and should then be encouraged to massage the scar with a moisturizing cream to improve its appearance and continue a healthy healing process. In the long term, massaging scars can prevent thickening and shrinkage of wounds.

Facial fractures (see also Chapter 11)

Fractures in children are characterized by rapid healing and rapid remodelling. In many ways these fractures are easy to treat and have minimal complications. In most such fractures reduction and fixation are not necessary. If fixation is required, *microplating systems* are normally used, as they are less bulky than miniplates. In intracapsular mandibular condyle fractures there is a risk of ankylosis, and early mobilization is necessary. Where fracture lines pass each other through unerupted teeth, there is an increased risk of developmental abnormalities in the tooth or early tooth loss.

Children who have sustained facial fractures require immediate assessment of their injuries, and this should be managed in a systematic manner. Details of the accident and any emergency treatment given at the time of injury are noted. The nursing staff observe the child's condition, appearance and vital signs, and then prioritize the care needed. When dealing with major facial fractures there is the potential for airway obstruction, and this is a major surgical and nursing consideration. Prompt and effective treatment can prevent airway obstruction from occurring. A full systematic examination is performed and any other injuries are identified. If the child has been involved in a road traffic accident they may have sustained other injuries that will take priority over any facial trauma. The priorities in children following multiple injuries are the same as those for adults. Facial fractures are often associated with head injury, and neurological status must be investigated and treated accordingly. Only when the child's condition is stable and other injuries manageable will the maxillofacial surgeon begin to manage the facial trauma. Facial fractures can also involve the orbit, and the visual acuity must be assessed (using a Snellon chart or pictures for younger children). Visual acuity and eye observations must continue post-operatively.

Children with facial fractures may present with very few symptoms. Whatever the plan of treatment, the surgeons and nursing staff will keep the child and their parents updated and informed. The pre-operative planning will be the same as for any other paediatric emergency admission, namely information and reassurance, care of the injured area, child and parental participation, and comfort and safety. At all times the child must be nursed upright in order to reduce the facial swelling. An intravenous infusion may be started if the child has difficulty in taking fluids orally, and this will keep the child hydrated during fasting periods and surgery. Appropriate analgesia must also be administered to keep the child comfortable.

Post-operatively the child should be nursed in an upright position as soon as anaesthetic recovery allows. This will help to reduce facial swelling, which can be quite upsetting for the child and their family. Severe swelling can cause the child's eyes to close and this can be frightening. Ice-packs can also be used to reduce swelling if they are tolerated. Fluids and a soft diet can be introduced as they are tolerated, and any intravenous fluids discontinued. The child should commence oral hygiene as soon as possible, and must understand the importance of doing so. Mouthwashes should be used regularly, especially following food, and the child should be encouraged to continue normal tooth-brushing using a soft toothbrush.

The child's post-operative period should be pain-free and comfortable, with regular and appropriate administration of analgesics.

A post-surgery X-ray will be performed, and if all is satisfactory and the child is well they can be discharged. Discharge instructions must include the continuation of strict oral hygiene. All intra-oral sutures will be resorbable, and any skin sutures will be removed at 5–7 days.

Non-accidental injury

Any child presenting with a traumatic head and neck injury that does not appear to be consistent with the history given warrants further investigation. This includes injuries such as facial fractures, torn frenulum, bruising, abrasions, lacerations, puncture wounds and ocular trauma. When assessing children's injuries, sometimes abusive injuries can be fairly distinctive and obvious, while at other times they can be mistaken for accidental injuries. As nurses we need to get it right so that children are not being overlooked or wrongly identified as at risk of harm. Where there is certain and actual abuse, child protection procedures need to be started immediately. Where there is suspicion of abuse but some uncertainty exists, advice should be sought from a more experienced individual, either a paediatrician or a child protection advisor (or preferably both). A paediatric opinion should always be requested. Diagnosis can sometimes be difficult, but a number of factors have been identified that can be used to assess whether a child has sustained a non-accidental injury. The factors are not conclusive, nor are they diagnostic, and they should be used with caution. These factors should be used in conjunction with your own professional judgement and assessment.

- There may be a delay in seeking medical attention.
- The story or history given is vague and lacking in detail, the account may vary with every telling, and the accounts may differ from one person to another.
- The explanation and account of the accident are not consistent with the injury observed.
- The parent shows an inappropriate reaction to the severity of the injury.
- The parent's behaviour gives cause for concern, e.g. obvious signs of irritability and hostility, seldom touching or speaking to the child.
- The child appears fearful, withdrawn and sad, and avoids physical contact with their parents.
- There is disclosure of an abusive act.

This is not intended to be a prescriptive list, and the absence of one factor does not exclude the diagnosis of non-accidental injury.

Every nurse is morally and legally responsible for reporting any incidents where non-accidental injury is suspected.

Useful addresses

The Cleft Lip and Palate Association (CLAPA)
134 Buckingham Palace Road
London
SW1 9SA
Telephone 0171 824 8110

Changing Faces
1 & 2 Junction Mews
Paddington
London
W2 1PN
Telephone 0171 706 4232
Fax 0171 706 4234

Junior Let's Face It
Christine Piff
14 Fallowfield
Yateley
Surrey
GU17 7LW
Telephone 01252 879630
Fax 01252 872633

18 Altered body image

Michael Perry

'Mutilating' disease and surgery
Problems with communication
Psychological effects of orthognathic surgery
Preventing problems

Most people are prejudiced (i.e. readily form an opinion irrespective of the facts), some clearly more so than others, and we readily stereotype others on the basis of how they look, dress and act. Much has been written about how we perceive others and the links between 'attractiveness' and judgements of personality, ability, intelligence and social acceptance. The importance of facial appearance in development and social interactions has been shown to have an effect on the individual while they are as young as 3 months of age.

Such categorization can have its drawbacks, for with it goes a certain set of assumptions or predictions, none of which may be true. For example:

- 'professors are absent minded';
- 'blondes have more fun';
- 'the elderly are set in their ways';
- 'Chinese are superstitious'.

By fitting someone into a stereotyped category we perceive them as predictable and easier to deal with.

Furthermore, we often feel that 'beautiful' people are more likely to be kind, good, sociable, confident and successful. Some studies have shown that attractive people tend to have better jobs and social interactions, resulting in high self-esteem, ambition and success. Conversely we tend to 'shy away' from deformed or 'ugly' individuals and feel uncomfortable in their presence, even though we may know nothing about them. People with severe facial deformities may be avoided altogether, while those with milder deformities may be ridiculed and, especially when young, made fun of by their peers. In some cases this may result in patients developing antisocial behaviour. It is believed that stereotyping develops early in childhood and continues to be reinforced during adulthood.

The extent to which appearance affects individuals is unknown. However, it is considered to be an important factor in the development of self-esteem, successful interactions and overall behaviour. Facial alterations, either following orthognathic surgery or as a result of disease and its treatment, may therefore have an impact on the perceptions and expectations of both the patient and those around him or her. Both may be positive or negative.

'Mutilating' disease and surgery

Despite 'state of the art' reconstructive surgery and good clinical outcomes, many patients never fully regain their pre-morbid appearance and function, and may be frequently reminded of their losses, particularly if this involves surgery to the mouth or a sensory organ such as an eye. Loss of body parts can have several psychological consequences. These may occur as a result of changes in form – alterations in the way in which the patient and others perceive their body – or changes in function, e.g. alterations in activities such as speech and feeding. This is particularly apparent if dependancy ensues. Anxiety, depression and sexual problems are often seen, and patients may develop avoidance behaviour or an obsessive preoccupation with the loss.

Many similarities are observed between grief following such surgery and that following bereavement. These include:

- shock or disbelief;
- pining for what is lost – this can be very frustrating leading to irritability and anger;
- depression;
- acceptance, the extent of which varies with self-confidence as self-sufficiency improves.

Following extensive surgery, 'loss' can mean loss of physical attractiveness (body image), loss of function, or both. Many patients may experience difficulty in coming to terms with their loss and may avoid reminders of it.

Cancer and major craniofacial trauma may result in alterations of body image, impaired functions and threat to life itself. Fear and grief are therefore likely consequences. Coping mechanisms vary considerably from one patient to another and may be partly related to the way in which they feel that the disease or its treatment has made them different to others. Radiotherapy that results in loss of hair, dry mouth, etc., can lead to further loss of self-esteem, grief and depression. In addition, the patient may still be anxious that the cancer itself has not been completely removed. Studies of patients undergoing breast surgery have shown that, although limited resection may in some cases be less psychologically dramatic than mastectomy, in others it is associated with a higher incidence of anxiety and depression due to fear of recurrence of the disease.

Problems with communication

Patients with communication problems following surgery often feel that they have become a burden to all who encounter them. Depression and feelings of worthlessness are also common, and are often made worse when no attempt is made by others to try to establish a rapport (the so-called 'does he take sugar?' syndrome). As a result, they may give up trying to cope with their disability. However, in most cases communication in some form or other is always possible, and with time a great deal can be achieved. Most patients are reassured to know that we can understand them even if there is no way in which we can change their circumstances.

Psychological effects of orthognathic surgery

Several studies have suggested that:

- physical attraction is important in the development of 'self-concept';
- physically attractive people receive more positive social feedback, reinforcing their positive self-image;
- 'unattractive' people often develop a negative self-image and even poor mental health;
- in *selected* cases surgical intervention can enhance physical appearance, which can in turn improve self-confidence and psychological well-being.

One of the most important aspects of assessing patients for surgery is determining those who may positively benefit from it. Defining what is 'attractive' and what is not is highly subjective. Although models are available based on the 'ideal' face, not everyone may agree with these features. Furthermore, racial and ethnic factors also need to be taken into account. Cosmetic surgery is a potential minefield, and thorough evaluation, often including psychological profiling, is essential. Despite the potential pitfalls, many studies have reported an increase in self-confidence in 50–75 per cent of patients following orthognathic surgery. One interesting study suggested that:

- some physical defects may contribute to criminal behaviour;
- in some prisoners cosmetic correction improves behaviour and helps to increase confidence about re-entry into society;
- if some deformities can be corrected early in life, young delinquents may avoid becoming criminal.

Other studies, particularly in rhinoplasty patients, have also shown positive changes following surgery. However, very often the degree of psychiatric improvement is unrelated to the degree of initial deformity. What is important is what the patient perceives to be abnormal. Even patients with minimal imperfections can benefit from surgery, and in some cases may exhibit less aggression, agitation and depression.

Preventing problems

Counselling, with emotional support and the opportunity to discuss concerns, reduces the prevalence of psychological problems after mutilating surgery. Patients should have realistic expectations of what can be achieved. They may develop anxieties in the form of both hope and dread. Further measures may include relaxation techniques, and in selected cases patients may benefit from medication. When there are clinical indications, depressed patients can be prescribed antidepressant medication. Clinical psychologists have much to offer such patients.

In most cases of malignancy it should be possible to prepare patients when they are going to lose tissue. This will reduce the shock when it actually happens. In the long term, most patients and their relatives appreciate frankness and openness about a poor prognosis. When appropriate, it is also important for professionals to be quite clear about the futility of undertaking wasteful treatments.

Patients need the opportunity to grieve, and for this to be acknowledged as a normal reaction and not a sign that they are breaking down. Members of the family also need these opportunities. Many of them wish to be involved in the rehabilitation process from the start, so that they can become part of the rehabilitation team once the patient is discharged.

Glossary

Accessory nerve The eleventh cranial nerve, the motor supply to trapezius and sternomastoid muscles.

Aerodigestive Relating to the upper respiratory and digestive tracts.

Afferent Relating to sensory nerve fibres.

Alar dome The bulbous tip of the nose.

Albinism Congenital defect in which the body fails to produce the protective skin pigment, melanin.

Allodynia The sensation of pain caused by a stimulus that normally would not produce pain.

Alveolus Tooth-supporting bone.

Anarthria An inability to move any speech musculature.

Angio- Relating to blood vessels.

Ankylosis Abnormal fusion across a joint space thereby reducing mobility. It can be fibrous or bony.

Anterior open bite When in occlusion (teeth together) only the posterior teeth meet. There is a gap between the upper and lower incisors, hence 'open' bite.

Antrum The maxillary sinus.

Apex The tip of the root where blood vessels enter the pulp.

Aphasia Total loss of language function, rendering the patient incapable of understanding speech, reading, speaking or writing.

Aphonia Voicelessness, due to paralysed vocal folds, laryngectomy or tracheostomy cuff inflation.

Apicectomy Surgical removal of the tip(s) of the root of a tooth, usually in preparation for a root filling.

Avulsed Traumatically pulled out.

Axial flap A flap of skin/muscle in which the blood supply is dependent on a single artery running through the pedicle (e.g. pectoralis major flap).

Barotrauma Injury as a result of high atmospheric/gas pressure.

Battle's sign Bruising around the mastoid process, which may represent a fracture of the skull base.

Bruxism Clenching or grinding of the teeth.

Buccal fat pad Fatty tissue in the cheek.

Cachexia Weight loss associated with cancer.

Calvarium Vault of the skull.

Cancellous bone 'Inner' bone sandwiched between outer cortical bone.

Canthi 'Corners' of the eye.

Carcinogens Substances believed to cause cancer (e.g. tobacco, alcohol and ultraviolet light).

Chemosis Oedema of the conjunctiva.

Chyle The milky-white fatty fluid absorbed from the gut during digestion. It enters the circulation via the thoracic duct or right lymphatic duct at the base of the neck.

Columella When viewed from below this is the tissue that separates the nasal airways.

Commensal organisms Organisms that are normally found on healthy tissues, many of which exist in the mouth.

Comminuted Multiple (more than two) fragments.

Compound The fracture overlying skin/mucosa is breached, allowing organisms to enter the fracture.

Condyle The head of the mandible which articulates with the base of the skull (articular fossa).

Cortical bone Thick 'outer' or surface bone.

Costochondral graft Rib/costal cartilage graft often used in reconstruction of the TMJ.

CPAP Continuous positive airway pressure.

Craniotomy Removal of part of the skull (cranium) to gain access to the deeper structures (e.g. brain, skull base, orbital roof).

Crepitus A crackling sensation caused either by the rubbing together of fractured bone ends or by air in the soft tissues.

Cupid's bow The bow shape formed by the vermilion/skin junction in the upper lip.

Cyst Fluid-filled sac.

DDAVP (desmopressin) A compound used to boost factor VII levels temporarily in mild to moderate haemophiliacs (see BNF).

Dead space A potential space or cavity which may be present following removal of tissue (tumour, cyst), in which blood and other fluids may collect, stagnate and become infected.

Decompensate To place teeth in their 'ideal' position within the arch.

Dehiscence Wound breakdown.

Dermatome The area of skin supplied by a single spinal sensory root.

Diplopia Double vision.

Dysaesthesia Dullness of sensation or the sensation of pain caused by a stimulus that would not normally produce pain.

Dysarthria Slurred, indistinct speech due to impaired speech musculature that affects articulation, resonance and intelligibility.

Dysphagia Difficulty in swallowing.

Dysphasia Disturbance of language function centred in the temporo-parietal region of the left hemisphere. This results in difficulty in finding words, understanding speech, reading and writing, and it is usually the result of a stroke or head injury.

Dysphonia Voice impairment, usually affecting vocal quality and loudness. This results in huskiness, croakiness, weakness and disorders of nasal resonance hypernasality. May be seen in cleft palate speech or hyponasality (e.g. from enlarged adenoids).

Dyspraxia Inability to perform a voluntary movement in the absence of paralysis.

Ecchymosis Bruise.

-ectomy Surgical removal of an organ (e.g. appendicectomy, cholecystectomy, parotidectomy).

Ectopic Abnormal position (e.g. fetus, tooth).

Edentulous Toothless.

Elective Routine.

Enophthalmous 'Sinking' back of the eye in the orbit.

Epistaxis Nosebleed.

Erythroplakia A red patch or plaque that cannot be characterized clinically or pathologically as any other condition.

Eschar A 'scab'.

Euthyroid The condition in which the thyroid gland is neither over- nor underactive, i.e. within the normal range clinically or biochemically.

Exostoses A localized abnormal bony swelling.

Extirpation (of pulp) Complete removal of the pulp of a tooth.

Facial nerve The seventh cranial nerve. Its fibres include the motor supply to the muscles of facial expression and taste fibres from the tongue.

Fauces The upper part of the throat, including the space surrounded by the palate, back of the tongue, tonsils, adenoids, palatoglossus and palatalpharyngeus muscles.

Fistula An abnormal communication between two epithelial lined surfaces, e.g. arteriovenous fistula or parotid salivary fistula (the communication that develops following trauma, surgery or pathology between the duct system of a salivary gland and the skin).

Gingiva 'Gums'.

Glossus Relating to the tongue.

Glossectomy Excision of part or all of the tongue.

Gnathic Relating to the jaws.

Gorling Goltz syndrome A hereditary condition with multiple features including multiple and recurrent basal-cell carcinomas (BCCs) and odontogenic keratocysts of the jaws.

-gram Radiographic picture using contrast medium, e.g. sialogram (imaging of the duct system of salivary glands).

Granuloma A nodule of granulation tissue (immature capillary loops and connective tissue).

Gunning splints Devices used to splint edentulous mandibles. They are similar in appearance to , except that the teeth are replaced by interlocking surfaces which enable the jaws to be held together in a similar way to IMF. Gunnings splints are secured by passing wires around the upper and lower jaws.

Hyperbaric oxygen therapy Treatment in which oxygen is breathed under pressure in hyperbaric chambers. Patients undergo a number of 'dives' as part of a protocol in specialist units. It is often used in the management of osteoradionecrosis.

Hyperplasia An excess of tissue (increased number of cells).

Hyphema Blood in the anterior chamber of the eye.

Hypo- Deficiency or lack/below or beneath.

Hypoplasia A deficiency of tissue (reduced number of cells).

Hypertrophy An excess of tissue (increased size of cells).

Idiopathic Cause unknown.

Impacted Relating to the situation where the path of eruption of a tooth is obstructed by another tooth, cyst or other pathology, commonly seen in wisdom teeth.

In extremis With a condition that is so severe that the patient will die if immediate action is not taken.

Infra-occlusion A tooth or teeth that do not erupt fully and lie at a lower level than the crowns of the rest in the 'occlusal plane'.

INR International Normalized Ratio, used to measure blood clotting.

Intercanthal distance The distance between the inner 'corners' of the eyes (canthi), often quoted to be around 33–35 mm.

Ipsilateral On the same side.

Keratoconjunctivitis sicca Inflammation of the cornea and conjunctiva (associated with Sjögrens disease).

Leukoplakia A white patch that cannot be characterized clinically or histologically as any other disease, and that is not associated with any physical or chemical agents except tobacco.

Lith A stone, e.g. sialolith (a stone in a salivary gland).

Meningoencephaloceles Herniation of the brain and meninges.

Mesodermal Relating to immature connective tissues.

Microcephaly Abnormally small head.

Microleakage Leakage occurring at a microscopic level, often around inadequate or longstanding fillings.

Midryasis Dilation of the pupil.

Morbidity Any complication(s) (except death) following treatment.

Neural crest A structure that appears in the early embryo, from which the central nervous system, adrenal medulla and melanocytes arise.

Neuropathic Injury or disease arising from an imperfect part of the nervous system (e.g. neuropathic skin ulcers).

Obtunded With altered level of consciousness.

Obturator A prosthesis designed to fill or 'obturate' a cavity (e.g. maxillary obturator used following maxillectomy).

Occlusal plane The plane formed by the biting or 'occlusal' surfaces of the teeth, when the upper and lower teeth bite together.

Onlay A material placed on bone to augment its surface.

Operculum The flap of skin overlying the crown of a partially erupted tooth (usually a wisdom tooth). Food debris can collect underneath this and become infected, resulting in pericoronitis.

Oropharynx The region formed by the back of the mouth and the pharynx.

Orthopnoea Breathlessness on lying flat.

-oscope An instrument for looking into the body, e.g. arthoroscope (for TMJ).

Osseo-integrated Biological integration between a foreign material (e.g. titanium) and bone.

Osteoradionecrosis Death of bone following irradiation.

Osteotomy Surgical division of bone, which may be undertaken to reposition bones (e.g. malar osteotomy, sagittal-split osteotomy, Le Fort I osteotomy) or to provide access to deep stuctures (e.g. mandibulotomy).

Osteum A small opening in bone, leading to one of the sinuses.

-ostomy An artificial opening between two conduits, or between a conduit and the environment (e.g. tracheostomy).

-otomy Cutting something open (e.g. sphincterotomy, craniotomy).

Overbite The degree of vertical overlap between the upper and lower incisors when biting together.

Palpable fissures The gap between upper and lower eyelids when they are open.

Parenteral nutrition Feeding directly into the bloodstream rather than through the gut.

Paroxysmal nocturnal dyspnoea Sudden episodes of breathlessness that occur at night.

Per Going through a structure (e.g. percutaneous tracheostomy).

Periapical granuloma Chronically inflamed tissue at a root tip.

-plasty Refashioning of something (e.g. sphincteroplasty, rhinoplasty).

Plication Folded, plaited or hitched.

Pneumonitis Inflammation of the lungs.

Post-nasal drip A sensation of dripping at the back of the nose, often seen in sinusitis, particularly at night when the patient lies down. As the sinuses 'clear', secretions drain back under gravity, where they are usually swallowed.

Pre-auricular In front of the ear.

Premaxilla This refers to the anterior part of the maxilla which supports the upper central and lateral incisors (usually the front four teeth).

Primary site The site from which tumours originate.

Primary surgery Surgery to minimize the resulting deformity. This is indicated when deficient development of an abnormal part interferes with the development of associated normal parts.

Proclined Forward tipping of the crowns of incisor teeth.

Prognathism A condition in which the mandible projects too far forward.

Proptosis Forward positioning of the eye, resulting in a 'bulging' appearance.

Ptyalism Salivation.

Ramus The vertical part of the mandible.

Random pattern flaps Flaps of skin/muscle in which the blood supply depends on numerous mostly unnamed blood vessels.

Retinoids Compounds that are biochemically similar to vitamin A.

Retrognathism A condition in which the mandible is relatively too small, with loss of chin projection when viewed from the side.

Retrograde root filling The procedure when, following apicectomy, the root canal(s) of a tooth has a filling placed in it.

Secondary site The site to which tumours may initially spread (e.g. lymph nodes).

Secondary surgery Surgery to correct deformity which has arisen from previous surgery.

Sialocoele Abnormal swelling containing saliva.

Sinus Blind-ending tract opening on to a surface (e.g. pre-auricular sinus).

Sjögren's disease Autoimmune-based disease resulting in inflammation of the salivary glands and conjunctiva, often associated with rheumatoid arthritis.

Somatic Relating to the 'framework' of the body (skin, musculoskeletal, etc.), excluding the viscera.

Stomatitis Inflammation of the mouth.

Study models Dimensionally accurate models of the patient's teeth.

Subconjunctival haemorrhage Bleeding deep to the conjunctiva (i.e. over the 'white' of the eye.

Submucous fibrosis The deposition of fibrous tissue within the mucosa, particularly prevalent in areas of the world where chewing of betal quids is practised.

Sulci The natural grooves or depressions in soft tissues (e.g. cerebral sulci in the brain). In the mouth it refers to the grooves around the mandible or maxilla. Those between the bone and cheeks are vestibular sulci, while those between the mandible and tongue are lingual sulci.

Supernumerary teeth Extra teeth.

Syncope Fainting.

Synostoses Premature fusion of sutures.

Telangiectasia Small abnormally dilated vessels seen on the skin/mucosa, which may bleed.

Teratogens Substances believed to cause congenital malformations.

Tori Exostoses of the palate or mandible.

Trismus Inability to open the mouth fully as a result of muscle spasm.

Uvular The 'dangly' object hanging from the soft palate.

Velum Relating to the soft palate.

Vestibule That part of the mouth which is outside the teeth.

Wolf's law The law that refers to the remodelling of bone in response to forces applied to it.

Xeroderma pigmentosum A congenital defect in DNA repair enzymes.

Xerostomia Dry mouth.

References

Angaras, M.H., Brandberg, A., Falk, A. and Seeman, T. 1992: Comparison between saline and tap water for the cleaning of acute traumatic soft tissue wounds. *European Journal of Surgery* **158**, 347–50.

Appleton, J. and Machin, J. 1995: *Working with oral cancer*. Bicester: Winslow Press.

Brown, A.E. and Langdon J.D. 1995: Management of oral cancer. *Annals of the Royal College of Surgeons of England* **77**, 404–8.

Buckley, P.M. and MacFie, J. 1997: Enteral nutrition in critically ill patients – a review. *Care of the Critically Ill* **13**, 7–10.

Caunt, H. 1992: Reducing the psychological impact of postoperative pain. *British Journal of Nursing* **1**, 13–14, 17–19.

Cooper, D.M. 1990: Human wound assessment status report and implications for clinicians. *ACCN Clinical Issues* **1**, 553–6.

Cortis, J.D. 1997: Nutrition and the hospitalised patient: implications for nurses. *British Journal of Nursing* **6**(12), 666–7, 670–4.

Cutting, K. 1996: Managing wound infection. *Journal of Wound Care* **5**, 391–2.

Daeffler, R. 1981: Oral hygiene measures for patients with cancer. *Cancer Nursing* **4**, 29–35.

Dikeman, K. and Kazandjian, M. 1995: *Communication and swallowing management of tracheostomied and ventilator-dependent adults*. San Diego, CA: Singular Publishing Group.

Garrett, B. 1997: The proliferation and movement of cells during re-epithelialisation. *Journal of Wound Care* **6**(4), 174–7.

Groves, A.R. and Lawrence, J.C. 1986: Alginate dressings as donor site haemostat. *Annals of the Royal College of Surgeons of England* **68**, 27–8.

Hallet, N. 1984: Mouthcare. *Nursing Mirror* **159**, 31–3.

Harris, M. 1980: Tools for mouthcare. *Nursing Times* **276**, 340–42.

Hayward, J. 1975: *Information – a prescription against pain*. London: RCN Publications.

Henderson, V. 1960: *Basic principles of nursing care*. Geneva: International Council of Nurses.

Heritage, M. 1992: *Link nurses: a successful liaison*. London: Royal College of Speech and Language Therapists.

Heritage, M. 1994: *Dysphagia training for nursing staff*. Nottingham: Nottingham Community Health NHS Trust.

International Committee on Wound Management 1992: *Consensus Statement*. Brussels: International Committee on Wound Management.

Irvin, T.T. 1987: *The principles of wound healing*.

Jarvis, Galvin, Blair et al. 1987: How does calcium alginate achieve haemostasis in surgery? *Proceedings of the 11th International Congress on Thrombosis and Haemostasis* **58**, 50.

King's Fund 1992: *A positive approach to nutrition as treatment. A synopsis of the report published by the King's Fund Centre in January 1992*. London: King's Fund.

Laing, A.S.M. 1992: The applicability of a new sedation scale for intensive care. *Intensive and Critical Care Nursing* **8**, 149–52.

Logeman, J. 1983: *Evaluation and treatment of swallowing disorders.* San Diego, CA: College Hill Press.

Logeman, J. 1983: *Manual for the videofluorographic study of swallowing,* 2nd edn. Austin, TX: Pro-Ed.

Macleod-Clark, J. and Hockey, L. 1979: *Research for nursing.* Aylesbury: HM & M Publications.

Mallett, J. and Bailey, C. (eds) 1996: *The Royal Marsden NHS Trust manual of clinical nursing procedures,* 4th edn. Oxford: Blackwell Science.

Maurer, J. 1977: Providing optimal oral health. *Nursing Clinics of North America* **12**, 671–85.

Meers, P.D. 1981: Report of the National Survey of Infection in Hospitals. *Journal of Hospital Infections* **2**, 31–9.

Melzack, R. and Wall, P.D. 1965: Pain mechanisms: a new theory. *Science* **150**, 971–9.

NHS Executive 1997: *Augmented care period (ACP) dataset – intensive and high-dependency care data collection.* Leeds: NHS Executive.

Perlman, A. and Schulze-Delrieu, K. 1997: *Deglutition and its disorders.* San Diego, CA: Singular Publishing Group.

Royal College of Nursing 1996: *Statement on feeding and nutrition in hospitals.* London: Royal College of Nursing.

Royal College of Surgeons of England 1992: *Guidelines for day-case surgery.* London: Royal College of Surgeons.

Salter, M. 1988: *Altered body image. The nurse's role.* Chichester: John Wiley & Sons.

Seton Healthcare 1993: *Wound care today – tradition or innovation?* Oldham: Seton Healthcare Group.

Tomlinson, D. 1987: To clean or not to clean? *Nursing Times* **83**, 71–5.

Topham, J. 1994: What's new in wound treatment? – not a lot! *Journal of Tissue Viability* **4**, 86–9.

Torrance, C. 1990: Oral hygiene. *Surgical Nurse* **3**, 16–29.

Trenter Rothe and Creason 1986: Nurse-administered oral hygiene: is there a scientific basis? *Journal of Advanced Nursing* **11**, 323–31.

Turner, T.D. 1982: Which dressing and why? *Nursing Times* **78** (Suppl.) 1-3.

United Kingdom Central Council 1997: *UKCC says nurses have responsibility for the feeding of patients.* London: UKCC (press statements).

Wallace, E. 1994: Feeding the wound: nutrition and wound care. *British Journal of Nursing* **3**(13), 662–7.

Waterlow, J. 1995: *Waterlow pressure sore prevention/treatment policy.* Obtainable from Newtons, Curland, Taunton TA3 5SG.

Further reading

Banks, P. 1983: *Killey's fractures of the mandible*, 3rd edn. Oxford: Butterworth.

Bell, W.H. 1992: *Modern practice in orthognathic reconstructive surgery*. Philadelphia, PA: W.B. Saunders.

Bennet, G.F. 1994: Neuropathic pain. In Wall, P.D. and Melzack, R. (eds), *Textbook of pain*, 3rd edn. Edinburgh: Churchill Livingstone, 201–20.

Corsen, R.A., Langdon J.D. and Everson, J.W. 1996: *Surgical pathology of the mouth and jaws*. Oxford: Butterworth-Heinemann.

Dimitroulis, G. and Avery, B. 1994: *Maxillofacial injuries; a synopsis of basic injuries, diagnosis and management*. Oxford: Butterworth-Heinemann.

Dolin S.J. 1996: Trigeminal neuralgia. In Dolin, S., Padfield, N. and Pateman, J. (eds), *Pain clinic manual*. Oxford: Butterworth-Heinemann, 204–9.

Dudley, H., Carter D. and Russell R.C.G. 1992: *Robin Smith's operative surgery. Head and neck. Part I and Part II*. Oxford: Butterworth-Heinemann.

Girdler, N.M. 1997: Facial pain. In Dolin, S., Padfield, N. and Pateman, J. (eds), *Pain clinic manual*. Oxford: Butterworth-Heinemann, 82–100.

Joint Formulary Committee 1996–1998: *British National Formulary* No. 32. London: British Medical Association.

Wright, M. and Bennett, S. 1996: The intensive recovery concept. *Anaesthetic and Recovery Nurse. The Journal of the British Anaesthetic and Recovery Nurses Association* **2**, 12–13.

Index